LEARN MASSAGE IN A WEEKEND

NITYA LACROIX

Photography by Jo Foord

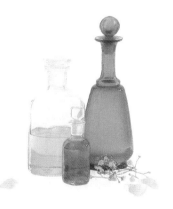

DORLING KINDERSLEY
London • New York • Stuttgart

A DORLING KINDERSLEY BOOK

Art Editor Alison Donovan
Editor Liz Wheeler
Series Art Editor Amanda Lunn
Series Editor Jo Weeks
Managing Art Editor Tina Vaughan
Managing Editor Sean Moore
Production Control Deborah Wehner, Helen Creeke

First published in Great Britain in 1992
by Dorling Kindersley Limited,
9 Henrietta Street, London WC2E 8PS

A CIP catalogue record for this book is available from the British Library

ISBN 0-86318-935-0

Computer page make-up by Cloud 9 Designs, Hampshire
Reproduced by Colourscan, Singapore
Printed and bound by Arnoldo Mondadori, Verona, Italy

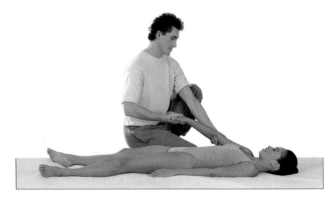

CONTENTS

·

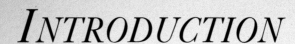

INTRODUCTION

MASSAGE HAS GROWN IN POPULARITY over recent years as its benefits are increasingly recognized as an antidote to stress-related problems – yet its origins are as old as mankind itself. People have always known instinctively how to touch each other in order to reassure, heal, and calm. As societies grew more sophisticated, this natural healing art was neglected. Now this is turning full circle, and more people are rediscovering massage as a means of achieving relaxation and wellbeing. Learning massage is a rewarding process, and will give you both a creative art and a technical skill, which you can share with your friends and family. In *Learn Massage in a Weekend*, I have presented the course in such a way that on the first day you practise each technique, learning how to create a sequence of strokes which you can adapt for different parts of the body. On the second day, you will use these skills in a series of specific massage programmes. This weekend is an introduction to massage, and some skills will need more practice to improve the rhythm, flow, technique, and intuitive responses that make massage such a wonderful experience for both giver and receiver. I hope you enjoy your weekend.

Nitya Lacroix

NITYA LACROIX

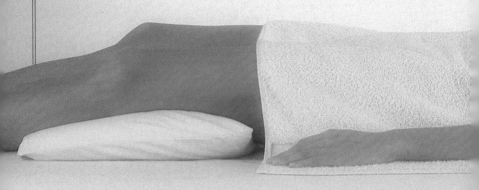

LAYING OF HANDS
Simple exercises of breathing and the "laying of hands", shown here, are integrated in this book with the more specific traditional massage skills. Awareness of breath, your whole attention, and the caring quality of your touch are as important as the actual techniques you are learning. In this way, your massage will reach the integral relationship between body and mind, to evoke changes in the whole person, and not just their body.

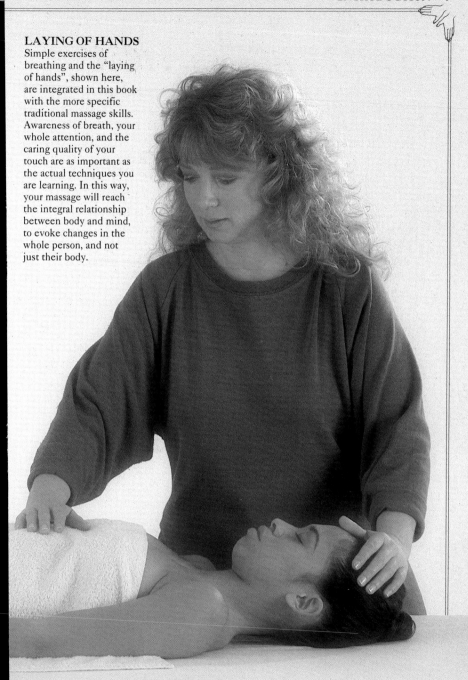

PREPARING FOR THE WEEKEND

Make your weekend a success with some simple preparation

MASSAGE IS MOST VALUABLE when the person giving it feels confident, and the person receiving it is relaxed. It takes time and practice to accomplish the techniques of massage, but with some preparation, you will gain maximum benefit from this weekend course. Choose a suitable place for your massage, equipped with everything you might need. Before you touch someone else's body, you should feel relaxed with your own, so try the exercises described to loosen up your body, to breathe deeply, and to energize your hands. Self-massage techniques will help

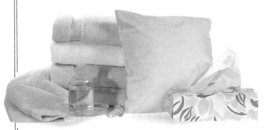

LIMBERING UP

Ease and suppleness enhance your ability to move about and apply the different techniques during massage. Limbering up exercises focus on your back to help you maintain spinal flexibility, and avoid accumulating tension (see pp.14-15).

ROOM AND EQUIPMENT

A comfortable and welcoming room (see pp.10-11), with the right equipment for both of your needs, will help you off to a good start. Warmth, light, and privacy are all important for relaxation, and you will need a stock of clean towels, sheets, and cushions.

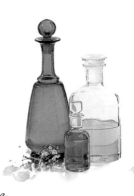

OILS AND STORAGE

The popularity of **aromatherapy** in recent years gives you a wide choice of **essential oils** to choose from if you wish to enhance your basic **carrier oils**. More specifically, you may like to try two simple blends for relaxation or rejuvenation. Storing your oils in suitable containers is important to preserve the oil's properties and to prevent it becoming rancid (see pp.10-11).

to get your hands in practice, and **postural** awareness will ensure you remain comfortable as you learn these skills to give your massage.
*Words in **bold** are given further explanation in the glossary (p.92).*

SELF MASSAGE
Practise the self-massage techniques to see how the strokes help to invigorate your own body, and to increase your hand dexterity (pp.20-21).

BREATHING
Deep and easy breathing (pp.16-17) is the key to staying relaxed yet energized. This vitality will impart itself to your partner during massage.

POSTURE
Good **posture** is essential while giving massage, if you are to enjoy the session and remain comfortable (see pp. 22-23).

CONTRA-INDICATIONS

Massage has many beneficial effects for health and wellbeing, and is an accepted therapy for stress-related problems and muscular tension. There are occasions, however, when massage should not be done without seeking medical advice first. Before starting the weekend course, or giving massage sessions subsequently, check the following list of contra-indications. If your friend, or client, has any of these conditions, do not proceed with a massage unless you receive the go-ahead from a doctor.
• Boils, skin infections, or any contagious or auto-infectious skin condition. Any area of skin that is inflamed.
• Avoid direct contact with areas where there is recent scar-tissue, undiagnosed lumps, varicose veins, acute inflammation, or bruising.
• Conditions such as cancer, epilepsy, Aids, or psychiatric illness.
• Acute back pain, severe injury, fever or a high temperature.

• Cardiovascular conditions such as thrombosis or phlebitis, or any other coronary disease.
• In situations of frailty, or pregnancy, or whenever there is any doubt about the advisability of massage, always consult a medical practitioner before proceeding.

AROMATHERAPY
Essential oils should never be taken internally, and instructions for dilution should be followed properly (see p.13). If you use essential oils in your massage treatments, you should consult a qualified aromatherapist about your choice of extracts and advisability of treatment, when working with the following conditions or situations, or whenever you are unsure about suitability of treatment.
• Pregnancy and breastfeeding; young children and babies; the elderly and frail.
• Epilepsy, high blood pressure or heart disease, cancer, and HIV-Aids cases.
• Asthma, allergy, or sensitive skins.

ROOM AND EQUIPMENT

What you need and how to prepare your room for massage

WARMTH, PRIVACY, SPACE, AND CLEANLINESS are basic elements in creating the right atmosphere, as you prepare your room and equipment for massage. Preheat the room, and maintain a temperature of at least 21°C (70°F), checking that there are no draughts. It is essential that your partner stays warm throughout, as body temperature drops quickly while lying still, particularly if the skin is covered with oil. A stock of clean sheets and towels should be placed close by to cover the mattress, and keep your partner warm and snug throughout. Decant your basic **carrier oil** into a suitable container, in addition to any **essential oils** that you may wish to use. Have a supply of tissues for wiping away excess oil. Keep cushions on hand for you to kneel and sit on, and also to be placed under your partner's body to ease physical tensions.

CUSHIONS AND TOWELS
Keep your cushions, pillows, towels, and sheets neatly piled up and within reach. Everything should be freshly washed, including pillow cases and cushion covers.

KEEP COVERED •
Use large towels to cover your partner so that he does not get chilled, and to help him feel more secure and less exposed. Remove them only when you are ready to massage the area.

PAPER TISSUES •
Excess oil can be wiped away with soft tissues. It is also good hygienic practice to wipe your hands clean after massaging the feet.

KEEP OIL AT HAND •
Place the oil bottle on a saucer for balance. You may wish to decant it into a squeezable plastic bottle, with a narrow neck or flip-top.

ROOM FOR RELAXATION

It is worthwhile spending some time on preparing the room, so that your massage area feels welcoming and comfortable for both you and your partner during your weekend of practice. Remove clutter as it will distract your attention, and make sure there is ample space to manoeuvre around the mattress. Choose a room where you know you can ensure privacy, and avoid interruption from your family, telephone, and doorbell. An open fireplace is inviting, and adds to the pleasure of the occasion in cold weather. Music can help you both relax, but choose carefully as it will affect your mood and the rhythm of the massage. Place your lamps so they cast a soothing light across the room, and try not to put the mattress directly below a bright bulb. Have your equipment neatly placed so that it is all within easy reach.

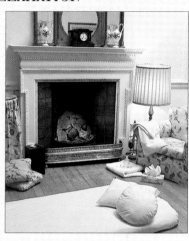

• BE CONFIDENT
Confidence is one of the most important aspects of massage. Good preparation will increase your assurance during the session.

LYING IN COMFORT

Your partner's comfort is paramount in your massage practice. Choose a firm mattress, futon, or foam rubber 5-8cm (2-3in) thick, for him to lie on, and cover it with a clean sheet. The base should be big enough for your partner, and also for you to sit or kneel as you massage. You could use cushions for your own ease, but do not kneel on a hard floor surface.

FOLDED TOWEL •
A towel will give a slight lift to the back of the head, and take the strain off the neck.

OILS

An introduction to the types of oil available that you may wish to use

OIL IS NEEDED as a lubricant during **soft tissue** massage, for smooth and flowing strokes. Your hands must be able to slide against the surface of the skin without friction. Talcum powder can be used as an alternative to oil, but this is not nearly as effective, especially for long, relaxing strokes. Cold-pressed vegetable oils make a good basic **carrier oil** for full-body massage, and have the benefit of bringing natural nutrients to the skin. Experiment with different oils to find the ones you like, avoiding those that are sticky or pungent. Popular oils are grape-seed, sunflower, safflower, and coconut. You can add a few teaspoons of the luxurious peach, avocado, or almond oils to enrich the mix, and a teaspoon of wheat-germ oil in your base will keep it from turning rancid.

CARRIER OILS •
Oils are of varying viscosity, so keep a selection of **carrier oils** so you have one suited to individual skin types.

• CORK
A well-fitting stopper prevents staleness, and helps to keep the **carrier oil** clean.

OIL RICH
For centuries, natural vegetable oils have been used to anoint, heal, and massage the body. Vitamin-rich vegetable oils are beneficial to the skin, and underlying tissue.

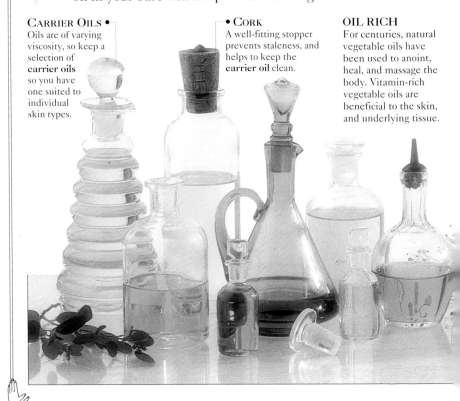

AROMATHERAPY

Aromatherapy is a healing art which uses the fragrant essential extracts of plants, flowers, and herbs to treat a wide range of physical and emotional conditions. The discernible benefits of aromatherapy have made the use of **essential oils** in massage popular, but it is important to know the exact properties and effects of each oil, and their contra-indications. If someone is being treated for a medical condition, (see "contra-indications" pp.8-9), or when working with the elderly, frail, and very young, check the suitability of your treatment with a qualified aromatherapist before you massage.

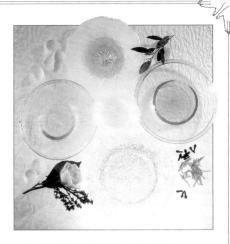

RECIPE FOR RELAXATION

Mix together: 7 drops of benzoin to warm and energize, 7 drops of lavender for analgesic effects, and 4 drops of camomile to soothe.

RECIPE FOR INVIGORATION

Mix together: 7 drops of rosemary for stimulation, 7 drops of rosewood for gentle uplifting, **grounding**, and **balancing** benefits, and 4 drops of basil to restore tired muscles.

MIXING SPECIFIC BLENDS

Essential oils are extremely concentrated and should always be diluted in a **carrier oil** before being applied to the skin, to avoid any allergic reaction. The usual blend is 3 drops of essential oil to a 5ml teaspoon of your basic oil. For sensitive skins, or when working on the very young or frail, use 1 drop per teaspoon. For a full body massage, you would mix approximately 18 drops of essential oil to 30ml of carrier oil. Mix only the amount you need for each massage and keep it contained in a glass or ceramic bowl, or easily poured glass bottle.

DARK GLASS •
Essential oils are extremely volatile, and need to be kept in dark glass bottles in a cool place. Never store in plastic in case of chemical interaction.

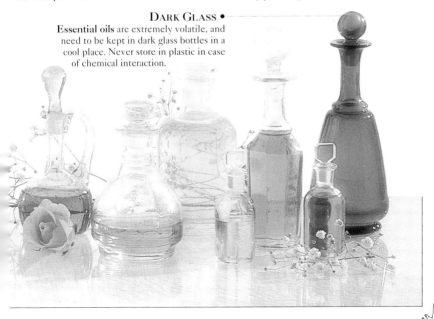

LIMBERING UP

Loosening up will enable you to give a better massage

FLEXIBILITY AND PHYSICAL EASE in your body are essential if you are to feel relaxed while giving a massage. Limber up your own body daily, or before and after the massage, to remain energetic and comfortable at all times. The fitter you feel, the easier it is to accomplish the techniques.

• ELBOW
Keep the elbow slightly flexed.

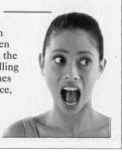

LOOSENING UP

These loosening-up exercises will help to ease discomfort and release tension gathered in some of the major joints of your body. The neck and shoulders, the face, and the spine are the areas of focus.

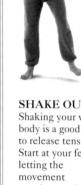

• FINGERTIPS
Shake your hands, to dispel tension out through your fingers.

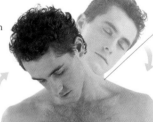

• PIVOT
The pivotal point is the top of your spine.

SHAKE OUT
Shaking your whole body is a good way to release tension. Start at your feet, letting the movement travel upwards.

NECK STRETCH
Circle your head slowly five times to the left and then five to the right, to give your neck a good stretch.

SHOULDERS
Circle each arm, slowly five times, behind your head and down again.

LOOSENING THE FACE

It is surprising how much muscular tension accumulates in the the face, particularly when concentrating. Emotional stress is also held in the facial tissues. Try loosening these areas by pulling some funny faces. This exercises and stretches the muscles. Begin by scrunching up your face, and then widen everything as much as possible. Pay particular attention to the areas around the eyes, mouth and jaw.

SPINE CARE

Your spine supports you. Its flexibility is vital to your health and wellbeing. Care of your spine requires regular exercise. These gentle movements help you stretch, flex, and extend your **vertebral column** and show you how to relax your whole back. A relaxed spine allows you to give a massage in comfort, without putting a strain on your muscles.

LOOSENING THE SPINE

Stretch your whole body upwards to the tips of your fingers. Hold the position for about ten seconds to feel the gentle pull in your back muscles, before flopping forward, so that your spine is loose and your fingertips brush the ground. After ten seconds, uncurl slowly upwards. Imagine each **vertebra** stacking individually.

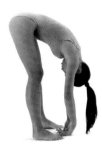
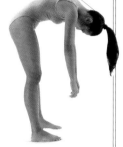

HEAD •
Bring your head up last, to balance easily over your spine.

FEET •
Place your feet about shoulder width apart.

• HEAD
Raise your head and neck, stretching the upper back.

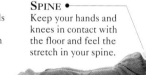

SPINAL STRETCH

Lie on the floor with your face down and your legs straight out together. Push up off the floor with your arms, raising your body until you feel the stretch in your lower back. Hold for ten seconds. Return slowly to the floor.

HANDS •
Keep your hands flat on the floor directly beneath your shoulders.

SPINE •
Keep your hands and knees in contact with the floor and feel the stretch in your spine.

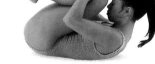

• KNEES
Bring your knees as close to your head as you can.

RELAXING

Below: After limbering up, take some time to let your whole body be still. Lay with your back flat to the floor, your legs and arms outstretched. Feel your entire weight drop downwards, and consciously relax your body, bit by bit, from feet to head.

CURLING UP

Above: Curling up takes the weight and pressure off your spine. Pull both knees up towards your chest and bring your head forward to meet them. Hold for ten seconds.

LOWER BACK •
Allow your lower back area to relax towards the floor.

Breath Awareness

Full breathing is the key to vitality and relaxation

FULL BREATHING unlocks your vital energy and helps to free tensions from your body. It also brings a release to both mental and emotional stress. Deep and steady breaths greatly enhance your ability to massage, by helping your concentration, and animating your strokes and the quality of your touch. Breathing supplies oxygen to the body, so it is important to breathe evenly while you massage. Encourage your partner to do the same. Correct breathing also helps to calm the mind and enhance attentiveness. Spend about 15 minutes on these exercises, sitting quietly until you feel you are in touch with your breathing.

Focus on Breath

Sit comfortably with eyes closed so that your whole attention focuses on your breathing. Become aware of the rhythm of each breath as you inhale and exhale, without forcing it.

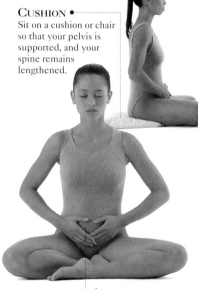

CUSHION •
Sit on a cushion or chair so that your pelvis is supported, and your spine remains lengthened.

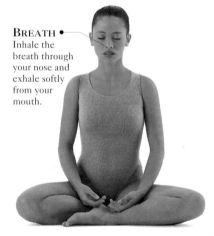

BREATH •
Inhale the breath through your nose and exhale softly from your mouth.

• ABDOMEN
Stay softly focused on this area.

ATTENTIVENESS
Rest your hands on your lap so that your palms are open and soft. If your mind wanders during this exercise, just return your attention back to your breath.

BELLY BREATHING
Breathing from the abdomen aids your vitality and stamina and relaxes emotional tension. Place your hands gently over your abdomen and become aware of their touch. Allow your breath to drop down into your belly so that you can feel it rising and falling. Relax the muscles with each exhalation.

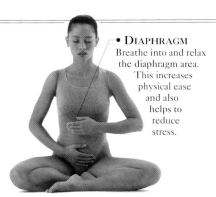

• DIAPHRAGM
Breathe into and relax
the diaphragm area.
This increases
physical ease
and also
helps to
reduce
stress.

• HEART
Imagine that the
area around your
heart is opening
up with the
warmth of
your hand
and each
breath.

SOLAR PLEXUS
Once you are breathing fully into the
abdomen, place your left hand gently over
the solar plexus area. Feel the rise and fall
of your breath in these muscles. Deeper
breathing in this area reduces anxiety and
increases circulation to all your vital organs.

BELLY AND HEART
The connection of breath between your belly
and heart is important. It helps you to relax
while massaging. Breathing deeply into the
chest, lung, and heart area enables you to
make contact with your own inner feelings,
and increase your awareness of this in others.

BREATH FLOW

Now you should be fully aware
of breath travelling through your
body. As you exhale, imagine
your breath is like a current of
warm air, streaming from your
abdomen, through your
heart and then out into
your arms and hands.
Enjoy this sensation
of full, flowing
breath and your
hands feeling
alive, receptive,
and warm.

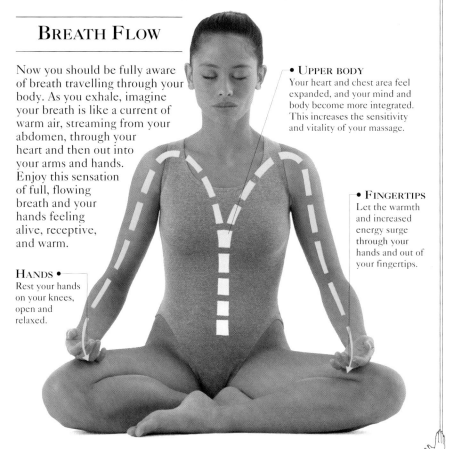

• UPPER BODY
Your heart and chest area feel
expanded, and your mind and
body become more integrated.
This increases the sensitivity
and vitality of your massage.

• FINGERTIPS
Let the warmth
and increased
energy surge
through your
hands and out of
your fingertips.

HANDS •
Rest your hands
on your knees,
open and
relaxed.

FOCUSING ON HANDS

How to use your hands to give a massage

ONE OF THE MOST important aspects of giving a good massage is the quality of your touch. Along with the technical ability to do the strokes, the dexterity of your hands and the feeling of warmth and energy that they can impart are intrinsic qualities. The hands should feel soft, vital, warm, and attentive to the body you are massaging. It is essential that they are supple, so they are able to yield to the structure of the body in the same way a potter's hands encompass and mould around his work. The breathing exercises on pages 16-17 will have helped to bring a feeling of life to your hands and vitality to your touch. Now it is important to get to know your hands better so that they can develop a confident touch, and be creative instruments with which you can share the medium of massage.

EXPLORING HANDS

Sit comfortably and raise your arms so that you can focus your attention on your hands. Look at them as if you are seeing them for the first time. Turn them from side to side to observe their size, shape, and shades of skin tone. Move your wrists and wiggle your fingers to feel their suppleness and flexibility.

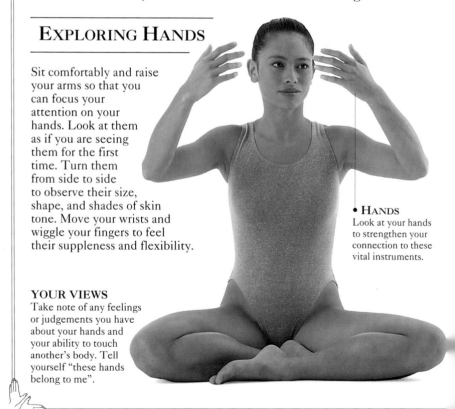

• **HANDS**
Look at your hands to strengthen your connection to these vital instruments.

YOUR VIEWS
Take note of any feelings or judgements you have about your hands and your ability to touch another's body. Tell yourself "these hands belong to me".

USING THE WHOLE HAND

Each part of your hand can be employed in massage, and your techniques will be more effective as your hands become supple and responsive to the different strokes and areas of the body. A flat hand produces a relaxed, flowing effect, while the palms are used for caressing, and reassuring movements. A light touch of the fingers creates a sensitive and pleasurable stroke. Heels, fingers, and thumbs, can penetrate a deeper level of tissue and release more tension from the muscles.

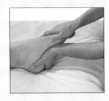

HEELS
The heels of the hands provide a broad, strong surface to ease away tension, and also stretch and manipulate tissue.

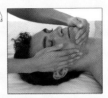

PALMS
The palms can be used to hold, stroke, and caress, helping your partner to let go of psychological and physical tensions.

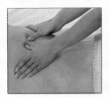

THUMBS
Thumb dexterity increases your range of strokes. Small areas of tissue can be penetrated, close to bones.

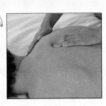

FINGERS
The fingers are good for a deep level of pressure on tense muscles, or a light, sensuous touch over the skin.

ENERGY BUILD-UP

Energy within the body is like electricity. The more that flows into your hands, the better your massage will be. These three exercises will show you how to increase that energy flow, bringing qualities of both strength and lightness to your hands. When you can feel an almost tangible sense of electricity in your hands, your strokes will become more effective. Practise these exercises until even your lightest touch will make contact with and relax the deepest recesses of the body and mind.

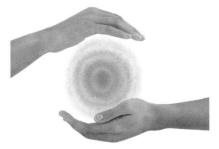

MAGNETIC FIELD
Bring the **breath flow** to your hands, palms facing. Slowly move your hands together and apart, so you feel a tangible force build up.

ENERGY BALL
With the magnetic field feeling dense and strong, use your imagination to shape it. Form it into a solid ball and feel its weight.

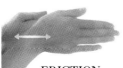

Repeat this exercise three times

FRICTION
Rub your hands together briskly for about 15 seconds. Stop and feel the heat and sensation of tingling.

SELF MASSAGE

Practise your strokes in a self-massage programme

BEFORE APPLYING STROKES to a partner, it is a good idea to practise them on yourself. In this way, you can start to experiment with different techniques, pressure, and touch in a way that is of benefit to your own body. It helps you build up confidence in your ability to use your hands and appreciate how good massage can feel. The strokes described here provide you with a simple range of techniques for working over all your body – from your head to your feet. Use them whenever you need to revitalize yourself or ease some tension from your muscles.

STROKING

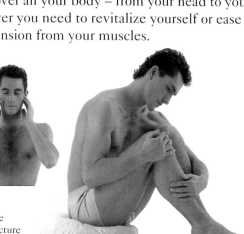

Lightly and smoothly stroke all over your body. First touch with your fingertips, and then your full hands.

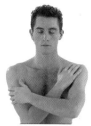

FACE
Above: Explore your bone structure and skin texture.

ARMS
Left: Stroke down your arms gently as if brushing out tension.

BODY
As you stroke over your body, mould your hands into the different contours and shapes. Try to let your hands "melt" into the body.

PUMMELLING

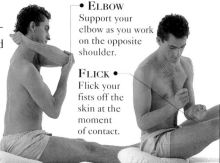

Pummelling the body increases blood circulation to the skin, and helps to relax tense muscles. Make loose fists, keeping your wrists relaxed. Gently pummel down your arm with one fist, starting from the top of your shoulders, working down to the hands. Then pummel over your thighs, using both hands rhythmically.

• ELBOW
Support your elbow as you work on the opposite shoulder.

FLICK •
Flick your fists off the skin at the moment of contact.

FRICTION RUBS

Friction rubs are a way to bring heat to the body, particularly over the vital organs. This works as a tonic to the system, restoring and boosting your energy levels. Place both hands flat on the body, and then rub them briskly in opposite directions. This friction generates a healthy heat.

KIDNEY WARMER
Give a good boost to your kidney area by applying vigorous friction to your middle back. Lean forward slightly for this stroke.

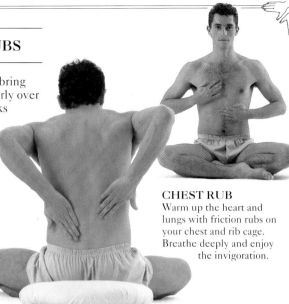

CHEST RUB
Warm up the heart and lungs with friction rubs on your chest and rib cage. Breathe deeply and enjoy the invigoration.

KNEADING AND SQUEEZING

Fleshy areas benefit from kneading and squeezing, which ease tense muscles, and tone up a sluggish system. Pick up and roll the flesh between your hands, giving it a firm squeeze. It feels great on arms and legs!

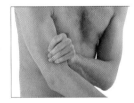

THIGHS
Fatty deposits can become trapped in the thighs, especially in women. Gently squeezing and kneading the fleshy muscles can help towards eliminating this, by breaking them down and increasing the blood circulation.

ARMS
Tension in the shoulders is often linked to tight, contracted muscles in the arms. Pick up the muscle between thumb and fingers and apply a firm, steady pressure.

PRESSING FEET

Feet often become sore and weary. Pressure on their soles, with thumbs, fingers, and knuckles can ease away the cramped feelings and create more space for the many small bones of their complex structure.

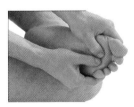

THUMB
Use both thumbs to press over the entire surface of the sole, one spot at a time.

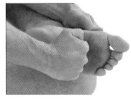

KNUCKLE
Using the soft edge of your knuckles, stretch the sole firmly from heel to toes.

TAKING CARE OF YOUR POSTURE

Hints for postural ease while giving a massage

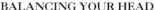

IT IS IMPORTANT to take good care of your **posture** while giving a massage. By doing so, you avoid undue stress on your own muscles while caring for someone else's body. A balanced posture will give your movements grace, help you to breathe deeply, and ensure that you complete the massage feeling refreshed. The chief objectives are to feel supported by your lower body, with your spine and neck lengthened, and not to overstretch, or hunch up your shoulders.

BALANCING YOUR HEAD

The weight of your head can put a lot of strain on your neck muscles if held incorrectly. Try to keep it balanced above the spine. A good tip is to imagine that the hair on the top of your head is being pulled gently upwards.

STROKES FROM ONE SIDE

When leaning over your partner from the side position, it is important to keep your balance. Kneel with your knees placed firmly apart, so that they can support the rest of your body. Always try to work directly in front of yourself, without twisting or straining your spine.

YOUR SPINE •
Keep your spine lengthened at all times. Avoid hunching your shoulders or bending over with your back. Relax any tension the moment you feel it.

UPPER BODY •
Keep your shoulders relaxed and wide, and your arms a little distance away from your body, as if you are wearing water wings. Keep your chest open.

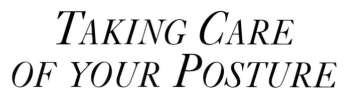

• **CUSHION**
When massaging the face, sit or kneel with a cushion comfortably supporting your pelvis.

• **HEAD**
If you lift the head or limbs, which can be heavy, remember to take care of your back.

STRADDLING

The straddling position enables you to work more comfortably on your partner's back. From this angle, you can apply long strokes directly in front of you with ease, without risk of twisting your spine, or overstretching your muscles. Straddle your partner by placing your knees either side of his hips. In this way, you will find it easy to add your body weight to your hands as you lean forward, increasing the pressure of your strokes.

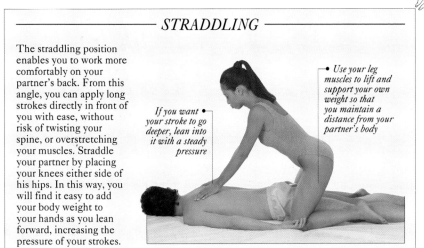

• If you want your stroke to go deeper, lean into it with a steady pressure

• Use your leg muscles to lift and support your own weight so that you maintain a distance from your partner's body

LONG STROKES
To accomplish long strokes, you need to move easily, without losing your balance. Place one foot on the ground with your knee raised.

• FOOT
To support this side kneeling position, keep one foot firmly on the ground.

SIT EASILY
Below: When massaging a small area like the feet, choose a comfortable sitting position. Support your spine with a cushion to tip your pelvis slightly forward.

LEVER UPWARDS
Above: Use your foot to lever your body forward as you reach into your stroke. Lean into your knees. To return the stroke, sink back down onto your haunches.

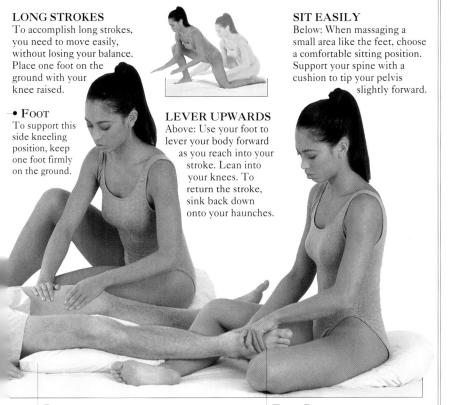

• PILLOW
Place a pillow under your partner's knees, to relax his **posture**.

• FOOT REST
Try resting your partner's foot on your own leg when working on the sole.

SUMMARY OF STROKES

The eight main strokes used in massage

THE EFFECTS OF A GOOD MASSAGE are both physically and
psychologically relaxing. At the same time it should invigorate the
system, boost a sluggish circulation, and assist in cleansing toxins
from the body. The techniques of massage, applied correctly, can
help relieve pain from tense, sore muscles caused by bad **posture**,
injury, or stress. Some strokes stimulate the **physiological** system,
while others enhance a feeling of calm and equilibrium. With
practice, a massage should bring a harmonious balance to body and
mind. Massage is a creative art. Learn the strokes and their effects,
and then trust in your hands to follow your own intuitive responses.

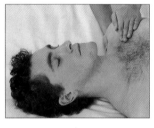

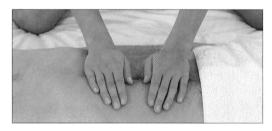

**POSTURAL EASE
STROKES**
Postural ease strokes will release
tension from joints between
major segments of the body,
such as the neck, shoulders, and
pelvis. Applied at the beginning
of a massage, they increase the
person's comfort in lying down.

ENERGY BALANCING
Energy balancing is similar to the healing techniques of
"laying on hands". These still, calm holds can be used at
any point during a massage, or as a complete session in
themselves. The purpose of energy balancing is to give
a sense of "**being** with" rather than "doing to" your
partner. With a caring touch, energy balancing holds
can impart deep relaxation within the body and mind,
allowing time for your partner to renew his resources.

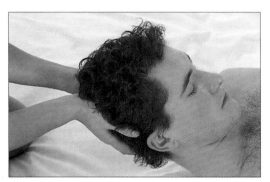

PASSIVE MOVEMENTS
Passive movements call for
confident hands for you to take
charge of your partner's body.
The aim is for you to take the
weight of various parts of the
body, such as the neck and head,
arms, and legs, and move them
without the assistance of the
person receiving the massage.
This encourages the receiver to
relinquish control in these often
tense areas, increasing a sense of
trust, letting-go, and relief.

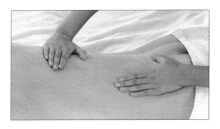
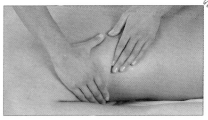

EFFLEURAGE

Effleurage, or stroking, uses the whole flat of the hand at a steady pressure in a smooth, flowing movement. It is used before and after all deeper strokes, and throughout the massage to integrate other more specific techniques. Hypnotic and deeply relaxing, it can also boost the body's circulation.

KNEADING

Kneading is an invigorating stroke, that helps to break down fatty deposits, and eliminate waste products at a deeper level. Muscles are manipulated by its rolling action, and the tissue's elasticity is increased. Kneading can be applied to the body's fleshy areas, and is a very satisfying stroke to receive.

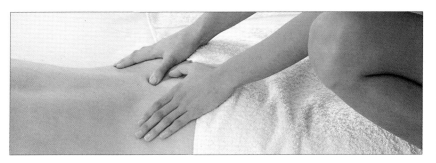

PETRISSAGE

Petrissage is a deeper pressure stroke, usually applied with the thumbs, fingers, or heels of the hand. It pushes the tissue towards the bone, and also helps to break down waste products in the muscles. After preparation with effleurage and kneading, petrissage can be used to create a firm, releasing stretch.

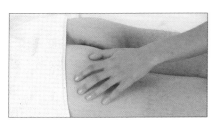
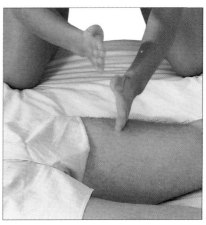

TAPOTEMENT

Tapotement has a stimulating and vibratory effect on the body. It shakes and loosens specific muscles by vibrating the fingers of one, or both hands, against a fleshy area. Tapotement can be used, for instance, on the cheeks of the face, the buttocks, or thighs.

PERCUSSION

There are a number of **percussion** strokes which revitalize and tone-up muscles. Rapid movements draw the circulation towards the skin. It is often used at the end of a massage to increase vitality. Percussion strokes include cupping, hacking, and pummelling.

THE WEEKEND COURSE

What you can expect from this weekend course

THE WEEKEND COURSE covers thirteen massage skills, teaching you the fundamental techniques of **soft tissue** massage. It shows you how to develop a confident, sensitive, and caring approach, to make the massage process a rewarding experience for both the receiver and giver. On the first day, the course teaches you basic massage movements and strokes, and shows you how to apply them in sequence. On the second day, this knowledge is used in a series of specific massage programmes. After the weekend, these elements can be combined to create a full body massage, so that you will be able to practise on your friends and family.

Hypnotic effleurage strokes (p.39)

Applying oil to your partner at the start of the massage (p.37)

DAY 1		Hours	Page
SKILL 1	Postural ease strokes	$1/2$	28
SKILL 2	Energy balancing	$1/2$	30
SKILL 3	Passive movements	$1/2$	34
SKILL 4	Starting a massage	$1/4$	36
SKILL 5	Effleurage	1	38
SKILL 6	Additional effleurage	$3/4$	46
SKILL 7	Kneading	1	50
SKILL 8	Petrissage	1	54
SKILL 9	Percussion	$1/2$	58

*Rest hold concluding the **energy balancing** session (pp.34-35)*

KEY TO SYMBOLS

CLOCKS
A small clock marks the start of each new skill. The blue section is a guide to how much time you may spend learning that skill, and the grey segment shows where the skill fits into your day. This does not indicate the time it will take you to apply any particular combination of strokes, but how much time you migh spend practising each skill until you feel confident.

RATING SYSTEM •••••
The complexity of a skill is rated by a one to five bullet system. Each massage skill combines technique with the degree of sensitivity and personal awareness brought to its application. Three bullets (•••) indicate that you can expect to achieve competency in the skill during the weekend course, while five bullets (•••••) mean that you may need to continue practising this skill after the weekend.

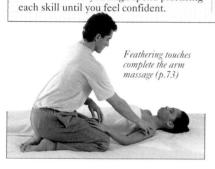

Feathering touches complete the arm massage (p.73)

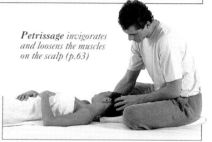

Petrissage invigorates and loosens the muscles on the scalp (p.63)

DAY 2		Hours	Page
SKILL 10	Massage for stress relief	1½	60
SKILL 11	Sensitive areas	1½	64
SKILL 12	Limbs	2	70
SKILL 13	Completing the session	1	78

Massaging for the relief of stress (p.60)

Helping your friend to rise at the end of the massage (p.79)

SKILL

DAY 1

1 POSTURAL EASE STROKES

Definition: *Bringing balance, comfort, and alignment to the body*

POSTURAL EASE STROKES are an excellent way to bring overall relaxation to the body before starting a massage. These movements stretch and release key areas of tension acquired by habitual poor posture. The person receiving the massage feels a sense of spaciousness in their body, and is able to lie down more comfortably.

OBJECTIVE: To help your partner into a lying position that is comfortable for receiving a massage. *Rating* •••

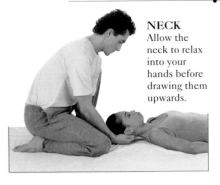

NECK
Allow the neck to relax into your hands before drawing them upwards.

EXTEND THE NECK

By relaxing muscular tension, the neck can extend upwards, freely. Slip your hands under the shoulders so that they are flat each side of the spine. Draw your hands steadily up behind the neck and out of the head. Lift the head slightly as your hands pass under the hairline.

OPEN THE SHOULDER

Bring a feeling of width and space to the chest and shoulder. Sandwich the shoulder between your hands, fingers pointing towards the centre. As you feel the area beginning to relax, pull both hands firmly and slowly out towards the edge of the shoulder.

ENCIRCLE
By enclosing the chest and shoulder with your hands, the whole area will start to relax.

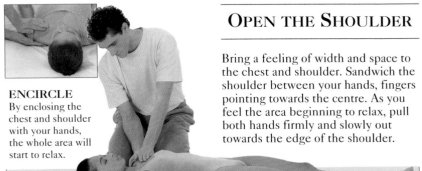

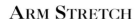

ARM STRETCH

This stretch creates a sense of length and release in the arm. Kneeling at your partner's hip, place your hands above and below the shoulder. Support the arm between both hands, and stretch downwards firmly, pulling the stroke out of your partner's hand.

CHANGE POSITION
You will need to change position to pull down the length of the arm. As a continuation of the previous stroke, this will release tension from the chest to the fingertips.

HIP AND LEG RELEASE

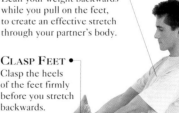

To ease tension from the pelvic area, slide your right hand behind the pelvis and your left hand under the inner thigh. Draw the top hand firmly behind the buttocks and then onto the upper leg. Give a stretch to the whole leg by supporting the limb with both hands, and pulling steadily downwards and out of the foot.

LEG •
To continue this long stretch, move your position further down the leg.

SLIDE
When the pelvic area relaxes, slide your hand down behind the buttocks.

PULLING ON FEET

LEAN BACK •
Lean your weight backwards while you pull on the feet, to create an effective stretch through your partner's body.

CLASP FEET •
Clasp the heels of the feet firmly before you stretch backwards.

Apply these **postural** ease strokes to both sides of the body. Now complete the whole sequence with an extra movement to give another gentle stretch to the hips and legs. Clasp both feet and pull them towards you, before slowly releasing your hold.

SKILL

2 ENERGY BALANCING

Definition: *Still holds effected by the "laying of hands"*

ENERGY BALANCING HOLDS bring essential feelings of stillness and equilibrium to massage. Use them as a session in themselves, or to introduce and integrate a massage. These holds are more effective if you close your eyes, and pay attention to your breath – allowing it to flow into your hands. Spend between 15 and 30 seconds on each.

OBJECTIVE: To assist physical and emotional relaxation. *Rating* ••••

HEAD HOLDS

These holds bring reassurance to your partner, helping to quieten an overactive mind. Use them to start or finish a massage, or while massaging the head, neck, and face.

CROWN HOLD
Your hands should be attentive and restful as you place them symmetrically around the crown of the head.

THUMBS •
Place your thumbs on the forehead.

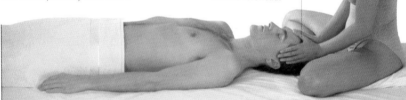

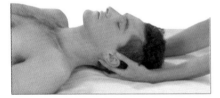

CRADLE HOLD
Place your middle fingers in the hollow area beneath the skull, right at the very top of the spine. Rest your fingers softly on the neck and place your thumbs beside the ears, to give a hold that is reassuring.

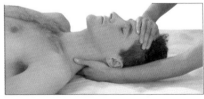

COMFORT HOLD
Resting your right hand gently across your partner's forehead, slide your left hand under the back of the neck supportively, with your hands pointing in opposite directions. This produces a very comforting hold.

HAND HOLD

By simply holding your partner's hand, you can impart a very real sense of caring. To create an even deeper feeling of relaxation and integration, you can then make a connection between the hand and the chest with one of these holds.

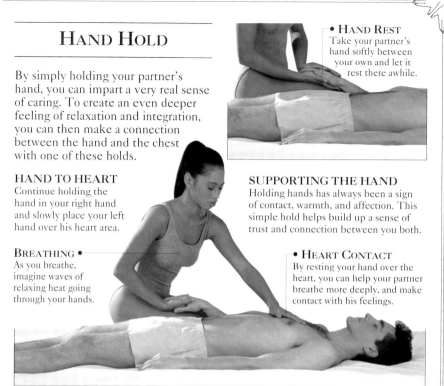

• HAND REST
Take your partner's hand softly between your own and let it rest there awhile.

HAND TO HEART
Continue holding the hand in your right hand and slowly place your left hand over his heart area.

BREATHING •
As you breathe, imagine waves of relaxing heat going through your hands.

SUPPORTING THE HAND
Holding hands has always been a sign of contact, warmth, and affection. This simple hold helps build up a sense of trust and connection between you both.

• HEART CONTACT
By resting your hand over the heart, you can help your partner breathe more deeply, and make contact with his feelings.

BELLY HOLDS

Emotional tension can cause the abdominal muscles to tighten. Your touch will help the belly to relax. Keep your left hand over the heart and place your right hand slowly over the belly.

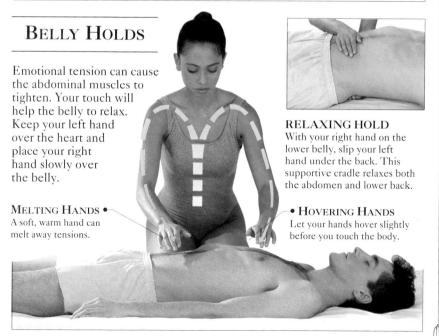

RELAXING HOLD
With your right hand on the lower belly, slip your left hand under the back. This supportive cradle relaxes both the abdomen and lower back.

MELTING HANDS •
A soft, warm hand can melt away tensions.

• HOVERING HANDS
Let your hands hover slightly before you touch the body.

SKILL

2

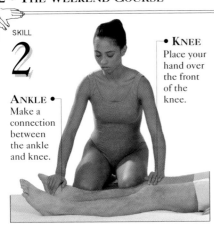

ANKLE •
Make a
connection
between
the ankle
and knee.

• **KNEE**
Place your
hand over
the front
of the
knee.

LOWER BODY

The lower limbs provide a system of
support and movement for the body's
physical structure. Ease within the
pelvis, hips, knees, ankles, and feet
creates a stable foundation for the
body and enhances good **posture**.
These holds bring warmth and
relaxation to taut areas, and provide
a sense of balance. Work down from
hip to foot on both legs, then back
up from foot to **sacrum** on the front.

KNEE TO ANKLE
The knee and ankle are vital in supporting
body structure. This hold eases away strain.

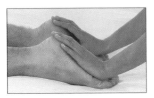

SOLE TO SOLE
Above: Holding the feet can
have a sedative effect, bringing
the conscious energy from an
overactive mind back down into
the body. It also balances the
left and right sides of the body.

FOOT TO SACRUM
Placing one hand on the
foot and the other on
the **sacrum** brings
your partner's
attention to
his lower
body.

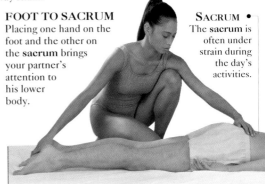

SACRUM •
The **sacrum** is
often under
strain during
the day's
activities.

— CONNECTION HOLDS —

Under stress, a person can feel
disunited in their body, or even
disconnected from some parts of it. One
of the most important elements of any
massage is to encourage a feeling of
integration and wholeness. **Energy
balancing** holds not only bring
harmony and equilibrium to the mind
and emotions, but can be used as
connection holds to do the same on a
physical level. After massaging one part
of the body, make a connection hold to
bring your partner's awareness to the
next. For instance, hold the **sacrum**
and connect with the knee or foot. In
this way your partner feels a connection
between the upper and lower body.
This promotes a wonderful sense of
wholeness and physical unity.

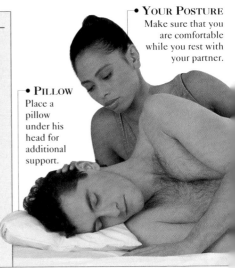

• **YOUR POSTURE**
Make sure that you
are comfortable
while you rest with
your partner.

• **PILLOW**
Place a
pillow
under his
head for
additional
support.

You do not have to follow any set format with **energy balancing**, but the sequence should be flowing and harmonious. Always work with the intention of creating a feeling of balance and integration within the body. Apart from following the examples shown here, trust your intuition, and place your hands wherever you feel your partner's body will benefit from their contact. Holds that are particularly effective are the ones which connect with major joints, and those that encourage relaxation and deeper breathing in sensitive areas like the chest and belly.

SPINAL HOLDS

The simplicity of this type of contact belies its beneficial effects on the body and mind. This is particularly evident when placing your hands over the spine. These calming holds can relax tension held deep in and around the spine, even with the minimum of touch. Hold your hands just above the spine before gently dropping them down on the **vertebrae**.

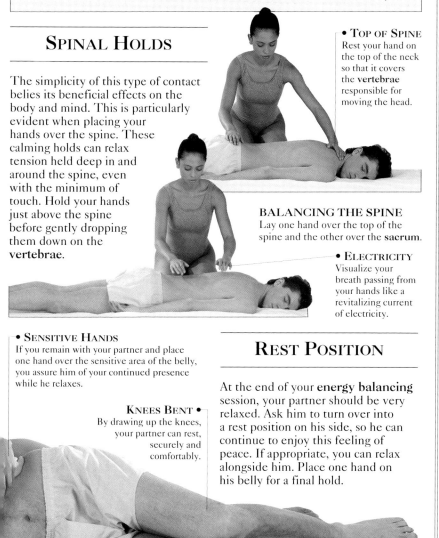

• TOP OF SPINE
Rest your hand on the top of the neck so that it covers the **vertebrae** responsible for moving the head.

BALANCING THE SPINE
Lay one hand over the top of the spine and the other over the **sacrum**.

• ELECTRICITY
Visualize your breath passing from your hands like a revitalizing current of electricity.

• SENSITIVE HANDS
If you remain with your partner and place one hand over the sensitive area of the belly, you assure him of your continued presence while he relaxes.

KNEES BENT •
By drawing up the knees, your partner can rest, securely and comfortably.

REST POSITION

At the end of your **energy balancing** session, your partner should be very relaxed. Ask him to turn over into a rest position on his side, so he can continue to enjoy this feeling of peace. If appropriate, you can relax alongside him. Place one hand on his belly for a final hold.

SKILL

3 PASSIVE MOVEMENTS

DAY 1

Definition: *A series of movements which stretch and relax the joints*

PASSIVE MOVEMENTS are effective stretches which loosen constricted joints. They encourage your partner to let go of rigid patterns of tension by allowing you to take complete charge. The art is to be confident and patient with your hands so that your partner can let go of habitual control, and relax while you lift, stretch, and take the full weight of parts of their body. Work down both sides of the body.

OBJECTIVE: To gain confidence in your ability to take charge. *Rating* ••••

RELEASING THE HEAD

Cup the back of the head, and take control so your partner feels safe

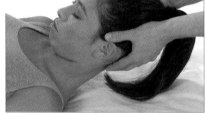

Anxiety, stress, and the heavy weight of the head can cause the neck muscles to tighten. By lifting and moving your partner's head while she remains passive, you can induce a deep sense of relief and relaxation.

The pivotal point is right at the top of the spine

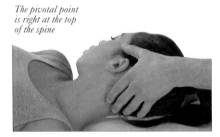

HEAD LIFT
Above: With the head in line with the spine, lift it slowly upwards to give the neck a full but gentle stretch. Lower it carefully back down to the mattress, so that its weight drops into your hands. If you feel your partner resist, or try to help the movement, pause for a moment. Repeat three times.

HEAD ROLL
Above: Once your partner has let you take charge of lifting and lowering her head, roll it from side to side to release tension from the base of her skull. Lift the head slightly and turn it to rest in your right palm while supporting it with your left hand, and then back in the opposite direction.

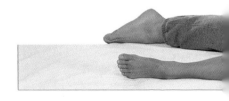

LIFTING THE LIMBS

The arms and legs are used a great deal in activity, support, and balance of the body. If the joints are stiff, their flexibility becomes inhibited. These passive movements help to increase their mobility.

PASSIVE ARM MOVEMENT

As you lift and lower the arm several times, the movement travels up to the shoulder joint and you should feel the arm becoming heavier and more relaxed. Swing the arm slowly out and back to the body.

• FLEXED ELBOW
Support the elbow, keeping it relaxed and flexed.

HAND •
Place one hand under the heel, to lever the leg upwards.

• KNEE
Keep the knee flexed. Support it by placing one hand underneath.

LIFTING THE LEG

Take care of your own **posture** while lifting and lowering the leg. As the leg relaxes in your hands, swing it slightly outwards to stretch the groin.

• YOUR POSITION
Lean your body weight forward into this stretch, keeping your foot firmly on the ground for balance.

HIP AND KNEE STRETCH

This passive movement flexes the hip and knee, easing tension from the whole leg. Use your right hand under the heel to lever the leg upwards, while your left hand slips on top of the knee to push it gently towards the body. This creates a deep stretch to the lower back, buttocks, and thigh. Pay attention to your partner's response to this stretch – do not push too hard, or beyond the point of resistance. Lower the leg smoothly back to the mattress.

• LEFT HAND
Slide your left hand over the top of the knee as you move the leg, so that you can push it gently towards the body. Ensure you keep the knee in line with the body.

SKILL

4 STARTING A MASSAGE

Definition: *The initial steps of a massage session*

THE BEGINNING OF A MASSAGE is one of its most important moments. It sets the tone for the whole session, and should create an atmosphere of trust which will enable your partner to relax more fully. Before you begin to apply the oil and strokes, you should endeavour to make him feel warm, comfortable and at ease.

OBJECTIVE: Giving your massage a relaxing start. *Rating* ••

Step 1
PUTTING AT EASE

Always ensure you have clean hands before you begin your massage. Welcome your partner. As he lies down, help him to relax by applying some **postural** ease strokes.

• KEEP WARM
Throughout the massage, cover the areas where you are not working, to maintain body temperature.

• ALLOW TIME
Give your partner some time to relax. Never rush into massage.

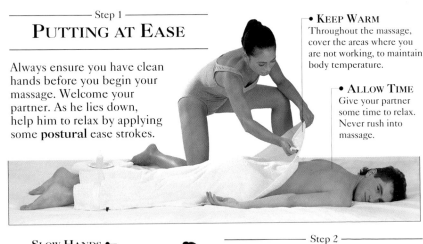

SLOW HANDS •
By moving your hands slowly towards the initial contact, your partner has less reason to feel defensive.

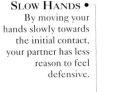

Step 2
THE FIRST APPROACH

As you settle yourself into position, make sure you have the oil close by. Take a few moments to breathe deeply so you can begin in a calm manner. When you feel ready, allow your hands to approach the body slowly and sensitively, as he may feel vulnerable and unsure of what to expect.

Step 3
THE INITIAL CONTACT

Begin the massage with an **energy balancing** hold. A still hold over the spine will help you both relax into this first touch, and make your partner aware of his back. Withdraw your hands slowly after a few moments.

• STILL HOLD
Try placing one hand over the back of his head and the other on his spine. Let your hands be still.

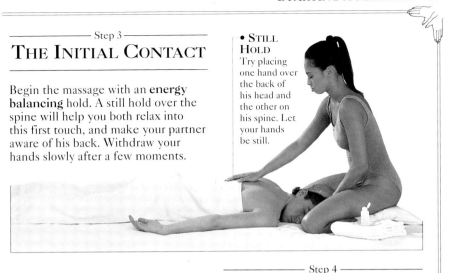

HOW MUCH OIL?
Initially, pour about a teaspoon of oil on your hands to spread over the body. Apply more oil if necessary – there should be enough oil on the skin to ensure a smooth stroke, but you will find that too much feels sticky and uncomfortable.

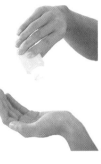

Step 4
SPREADING THE OIL

Now is the time to apply some oil to your hands. Squeeze it into the palm of one hand, taking care not to drip any onto your partner's body. Rub the oil into both hands, using this opportunity to warm them up. When they are feeling supple, start to spread the oil over the back of the body.

RELAXING STROKES
Take your time to apply the oil. These strokes over the back will help you both relax before you start to add specific techniques. Use this time for your hands to "pick up" any body messages, noting what areas feel tense, and will need special attention later in the massage.

• POSTURE
Spread the oil with smooth, flowing, and rounded strokes. From the start of the massage, take care of your own **posture**. Do not lean too far over your partner.

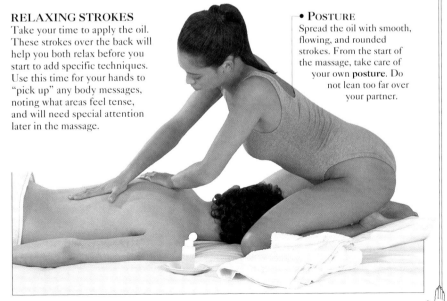

SKILL

5 EFFLEURAGE

Definition: *The smooth and relaxing basic strokes of massage*

EFFLEURAGE IS THE PRINCIPAL STROKE of massage. The strokes are smooth and flowing, and are applied with the flat of the hand at a steady pressure. Their chief effect is to create both physical and psychological relaxation. Effleurage moves and stretches the body's **soft tissue**, and helps to boost the cardiovascular system, especially when directed up towards the heart. Effleurage should always be applied before and after the deeper and more vigorous strokes.

OBJECTIVE: Learning to apply strokes which relax and integrate your techniques. *Rating* ••••

EFFLEURAGE AS A MAIN STROKE

*This skill shows you how to apply effleurage as a primary stroke over different areas of the body, to prepare it for your subsequent techniques. Never finish a **main stroke** abruptly, always round it off or take it right out of the body*

SLIDE •
The firm slide of your hands alongside the spine will stretch tense muscles.

BACK OF BODY

Place your hands either side of the spine at shoulder height. Slide them slowly down the long, supporting muscles, then continue by swinging them outwards at the base of the ribs.

• **HANDS**
Mould your hands into the sides of the ribcage.

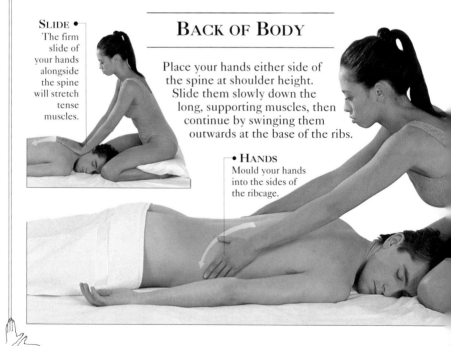

AROUND SHOULDERS

As you slide your hands up the sides of the ribcage and encompass the area, you will emphasize the symmetry of the body. When you reach the shoulder blades, flex your wrists so that your hands curve inwards, and slide them flat around and alongside the edges of the bone.

WRISTS FLEXED •
Flex your wrists so your hands leave the sides of the body.

SHOULDER BLADES
Once your hands have rounded the shoulder blades, pull them outwards over the band of muscles across the shoulders. Apply pressure with the heels of your hands.

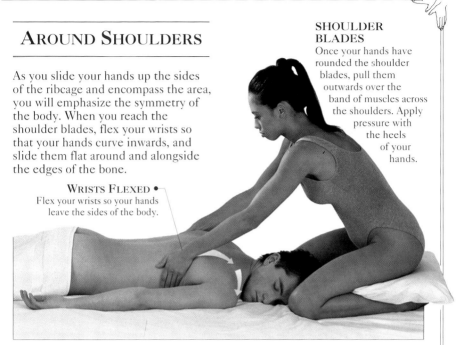

WRISTS •
Keep your wrists loose and your elbows flexed, so that they rotate around the shoulders easily.

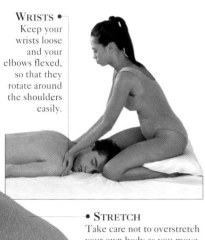

TOWARDS THE NECK
Left: When you reach the edges of the shoulders, lighten your pressure and swivel your hands to encircle the joints. Avoid dragging the shoulders up as you pull your hands towards the neck.

OUT OF THE NECK AND HEAD
Below: Once your hands reach the base of the neck, slide them up over it and out through the back of the head. Repeat the **main stroke** several times, and try experimenting with speed and pressure.

• STRETCH
Take care not to overstretch your own body as you move your hands towards the base of the spine.

MAIN MOVE
Left: While practising this **main stroke**, ask your partner for his comments on your pressure.

EASE TENSION •
This stroke eases tension from the back muscles. Increase the sense of relief by sweeping the stroke right out of the neck and head.

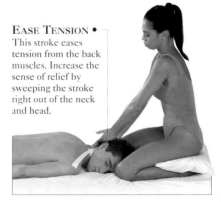

LEGS

*How to make the first **main strokes** on the back and the front of the legs*

BACK OF LEGS

The legs and pelvis take the strain of the body's weight. This **main stroke** warms, soothes, and stretches the whole of the leg, and prepares it for more specific techniques, as well as boosting a sluggish circulation with its upward sweep. Apply oil by stroking it down the leg, and then with your hands parallel over the back of the ankle, little fingers leading, glide them together up over the calf.

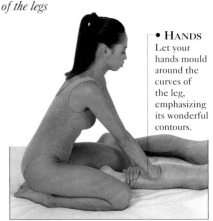

• HANDS
Let your hands mould around the curves of the leg, emphasizing its wonderful contours.

STROKING UP
Stroke up the leg, lessening pressure on the back of the knee. The leading hand slides around the hip, as your lower hand waits on the inner thigh.

• FLEXED HIP
Lean forward by bending from your hips.

• STILL HAND
Keep this hand still until the top hand has rounded over the buttocks, and returns to a parallel position on the outside thigh.

PULL DOWN
With both hands equally placed on the thigh, slip your fingers under the leg. Support the leg securely, and pull firmly back down the length.

• FINISH STROKE
When your hands reach the ankle, complete the stroke by sliding one hand under the front of the foot, and the other over the sole, to take the stroke right out of the foot.

COVER UP •
An oiled body quickly loses heat. To keep your partner warm, cover his upper body while working on his legs.

FRONT OF LEGS

The **main stroke** on the front of the legs is done in a similar way to the back of the leg, although you must take special care as your hands pass over the bones and joints, which are closer to the surface. Place your hands, little fingers leading, over the front of the ankle and slide them up the shin.

TAKE CARE
Right: The knee is a delicate area, so yield your hands softly around its bony shape.

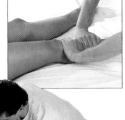

FRONT OF THIGH

Continue moving both hands up over the front of the thigh, feeling the muscles ripple beneath the stroke. At the top of the thigh, swing the upper hand around the pelvic girdle, over the hip and smoothly back down to the leg, while the lower hand waits on the inner thigh.

HAND •
The leading hand continues to stroke up and around the hip to ease tension from this joint.

THIGH STROKE

Separate your hands to encircle the full circumference of the upper thigh.

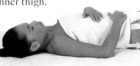

LEG STRETCH

When both hands are in the same position on the thigh, slide your fingers under the leg and draw your hands down to give a firm stretch. On reaching the ankle, swing your hands around so they slide out over the top and bottom of the foot.

YOUR LEGS •
Use your legs to manoeuvre back and forth. You will need to adjust your own position several times, to accomplish a long stroke like this.

GIVE SUPPORT •
Keep your hands steady and parallel, and in full support of the leg.

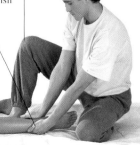

SKILL
5 THE TORSO

*These **main strokes** on the abdomen and chest prepare the torso
for your subsequent massage techniques*

THE BELLY

The basic effleurage stroke on the
belly is a circular motion. When you
are massaging the belly, remember
that there is no skeletal structure to
protect the vital organs here, and it is
natural for your partner to feel quite
protective of this part of her body. As
your partner relaxes, she will allow
your strokes to become deeper.

BEGIN CIRCLE
When your partner begins
to relax, start sliding the flat
of your hands slowly in a
clockwise motion on
the abdomen.

RIGHT HAND •
If you stand to your partner's
left, your right hand makes
a half-circle on the upper
abdomen before lifting off.

-*SENSITIVE APPROACH*-

Approach the belly slowly and gently. It
is a good idea to start with a calm **energy
balancing** hold, making a connection
between the upper and lower abdomen.
This will encourage your partner to
breathe more deeply, and start to relax.

Make the first •
*contact with
the area just
below the
ribcage*

• *Approach
the belly
area in
a calm
manner*

•**LEFT HAND**
The left hand makes complete
continuous clockwise circles,
following the natural movement
of the digestive processes.

MID-CIRCLE
When your left hand
approaches the
upper belly, lift the
right hand so the
left can continue
its circular motion.

LIFT OFF •
Raise your
right hand
slowly from
the abdomen.

COMPLETE
MOVEMENT
Once the left hand
has completed a
circle, continue the
strokes, deepening
your pressure.

RIGHT HAND •
Make a crescent
shape to emphasize
the last half of
the circle.

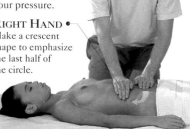

THE CHEST

When you massage the chest, you will feel that the skeletal structure of the ribcage is close to the surface. The **main stroke** on this area brings relief to constricted muscles connecting the ribs, and helps your partner to breathe more fully throughout the upper body. This will help to release both physical and emotional tensions.

CONNECT
Make a connection between the belly you have just massaged, and the heart area where you will now apply strokes.

STROKE UPWARDS
Start the main chest stroke by sliding both hands firmly up the breastbone at a steady pace.

FLAT HANDS •
Your hands should be flat, with fingers towards the head.

• POSITION
Kneel beside your partner's waistline and face towards the direction of your stroke.

• INTEGRATION
By keeping one hand on the belly, which is now relaxed, and placing the other on the chest, you enhance the sense of integration.

UPPER CHEST
When your hands reach the top of the breastbone, fan them out over the top of the chest towards the shoulders. This will release tension from the **pectorals** above the breasts, and bring a feeling of width to the shoulders. Continue sliding your hands around the shoulder joints.

PRESSURE •
When you repeat this stroke, try increasing the stretch by using pressure from your heels.

• BODY WEIGHT
Use your body weight rather than your muscles to increase the pressure.

FIRM HANDS •
Firm, soft hands will bring a feeling of shape and tone to the rounded contours of your partner's upper body.

RETURN THE STROKE
Slide your hands around the shoulders, down under the armpits and firmly along the sides of the body. At the base of the ribcage, flex your wrists and stroke lightly up to the breastbone. Repeat the stroke several times, in a continuous flow, taking care not to press the delicate breast tissue.

5

UPPER LIMBS

*This is a main effleurage stroke which covers the
full length of the arms*

UPWARD MOVE

Clasp your partner's hand to anchor the
arm, and avoid it being pushed up towards
the shoulder. With
little finger leading,
slide your other
hand firmly and
steadily up
the arm.

SHOULDERS AND ARMS

Arms are one of the most active areas
of the body, expressing both work and
creativity. Loose, flexible arms will
reduce tension in the shoulders and
add dexterity to the hands. This **main
stroke** relaxes the whole arm, warming
the skin, and prepares it
for deeper strokes. The
upward movement,
from the hand to the
shoulder, boosts both
the **lymphatic** and
blood circulation.

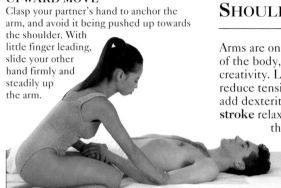

ENCIRCLE

Now release your
partner's hand to
bring your left hand
to the front of
the shoulder.

• HAND

This hand glides
over and behind
the shoulder,
encompassing
the joint.

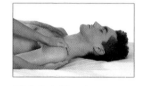

EMBRACE JOINT

Above: With both hands
embracing the shoulder,
begin to pull down the arm.
Your two hands should be
fully supporting the arm
as you give the joint a
firm but gentle stretch.

DOWNWARD STRETCH

With the arm securely held between
your hands, pull downwards
steadily. This will give a stretch
to the whole limb, and increase
the feeling of relaxation. Slide
the stroke out of the hand and
fingers. Repeat the stroke
several times, before
massaging the other arm.

• FLEXED ELBOW

As you slide your hands down the
arm, ensure your partner's elbow
remains slightly flexed. This will help
to prevent the weight of the arm from
locking the joint.

• RELEASE

A gentle pull at the
shoulder joint helps to
dispel pent-up tension.

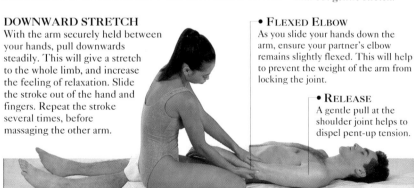

THE UPPER BODY

*A **main stroke** on the upper body, shoulders and neck from a position behind your partner's head*

STERNUM
Slide both hands down the breastbone, from top to bottom. Fan your hands out around the base of the ribcage.

PACE •
Your hands should maintain a smooth and steady pace.

RIBCAGE AND NECK

This main effleurage stroke is an excellent way to commence or bring to a close a front-of-the-body massage. It warms, relaxes, and soothes the taut areas of the torso and neck with its continuous rounded motion, while the stroke right out of the head draws tension away from the whole area. Practise this stroke until both of you feel satisfied with its beneficial effect.

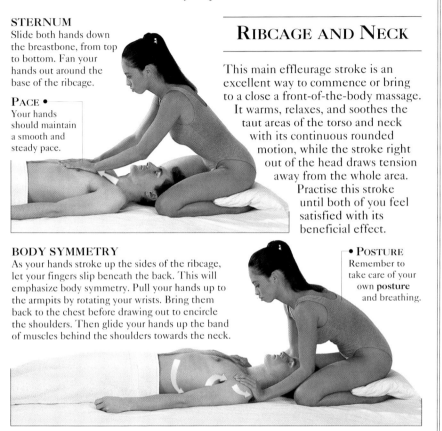

BODY SYMMETRY
As your hands stroke up the sides of the ribcage, let your fingers slip beneath the back. This will emphasize body symmetry. Pull your hands up to the armpits by rotating your wrists. Bring them back to the chest before drawing out to encircle the shoulders. Then glide your hands up the band of muscles behind the shoulders towards the neck.

• POSTURE
Remember to take care of your own **posture** and breathing.

RELEASE THE NECK
When the heels of your hands reach the base of the neck, swivel your fingers so they rest alongside the spine, pointing downwards. Give your partner time to relax his neck. Draw both hands steadily up the neck, firmly and confidently, to pull the stroke out through the back of the head. Lift the head slightly at the hairline as your hands slide under.

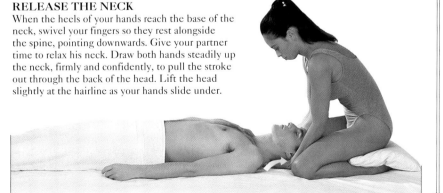

SKILL

6 ADDITIONAL EFFLEURAGE

Definition: *Soothing strokes that enhance mental and physical relaxation*

ONCE YOU HAVE APPLIED the main effleurage stroke, there are further **soft tissue** movements which will induce psychological relaxation, as well as soothe and stretch muscles in preparation for deeper and more invigorating work. This sequence shows you how to use them in a basic back massage, although many of the strokes can be used successfully on other parts of the body. After three flowing **main strokes**, from a position above your partner's head, move to his side. Circular and milking strokes should be applied on both sides of the body, so you will have to change your position.

OBJECTIVE: To learn more effleurage strokes. *Rating* •••••

FAN STROKES

Fan strokes are a lovely way to follow up the main movement on any part of the body. They are achieved by your hands making a restful, flowing fan shape. On the back, place both hands flat alongside each other, and glide them steadily upwards, then fan them out towards the sides of the body.

YOUR HANDS •
Begin by resting your hands at the base of the spine, and glide them up the back a short distance.

HAND PRESSURE •
Lean your body weight into the stroke to help you maintain a steady pressure as you slide your hands upwards.

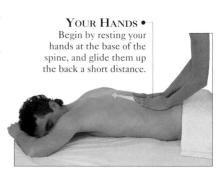

MOVING OUTWARDS
Above: As your hands fan out, soften their pressure. Encompass the sides of the body with a gentle squeeze, as your stroke draws down.

RETURN SOFTLY
Left: Swivel your wrists and glide back very lightly as you return to the source of the stroke. Let one stroke flow into the next, each time sliding a little higher up.

CIRCULAR STROKES

These are wonderful strokes that look simple, but need some practice to achieve their unbroken circular motion. They loosen up muscles on the surface of the back and sides of the ribcage. In principle, they are similar to the **main stroke** on the belly, applied in smaller circles. In these instructions, the left hand makes the complete circle, while the right hand makes a half-circle.

TO BEGIN
Place both hands parallel, a small distance apart on the side of the body. Start to slide both hands into a circular motion.

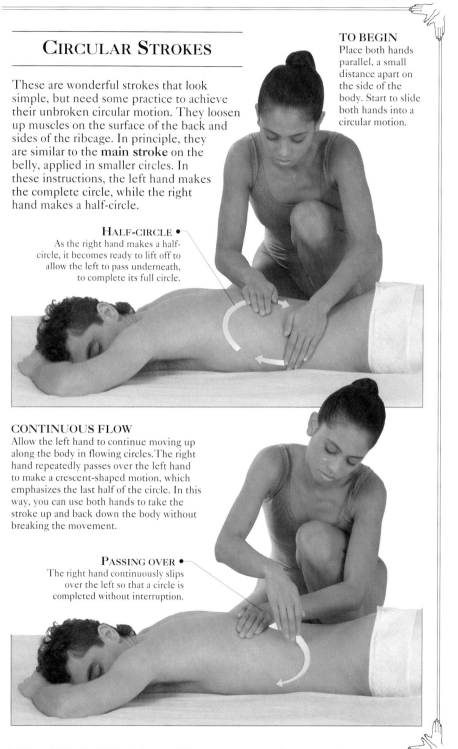

HALF-CIRCLE •
As the right hand makes a half-circle, it becomes ready to lift off to allow the left to pass underneath, to complete its full circle.

CONTINUOUS FLOW
Allow the left hand to continue moving up along the body in flowing circles. The right hand repeatedly passes over the left hand to make a crescent-shaped motion, which emphasizes the last half of the circle. In this way, you can use both hands to take the stroke up and back down the body without breaking the movement.

PASSING OVER •
The right hand continuously slips over the left so that a circle is completed without interruption.

SKILL 6

FINGERTIPS •
Slip your fingertips slightly under the front of the body.

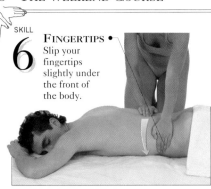

CROSS-OVER STROKES

Work these strokes continuously across the superficial muscle tissue, from the lower back up towards the shoulder blades and down again. They give a good stretch and gentle friction to the base and middle back. Begin by placing your hands flat over both sides of the back, ready to slide.

SWOP HANDS OVER
Both hands slide continuously past each other to swop from side to side.

• HEEL OF HAND
Glide the heel of your hand right down the side closest to you.

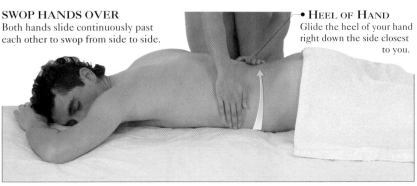

MILKING STROKES

Milking strokes focus on the muscles alongside the hips, abdomen, and ribs. Place both hands over the side furthest from you, ready to pull one hand after the other towards yourself. As each hand reaches the spine, lift it up and return it to the side, creating a continuous milking action.

UNDER BODY •
Pull your fingers from under the body to give the stroke a feeling of completeness.

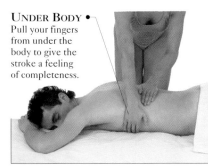

LIGHTEN PRESSURE
As your hand glides up on the back, lighten the pressure before lifting it off the body.

• RHYTHMIC HANDS
The hands should create a continuous rhythmic motion.

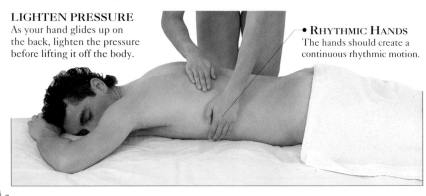

STRETCHING

Stretch strokes can introduce a feeling of play, as well as relieving areas of tension by adding a sense of length and width to the body. Stretching can be applied to the back, the sides of the body, and to the limbs. The flat of your hands move from a central point, in opposite directions, at a slow and steady pressure. On the back, stretch strokes can be done from the centre of the spine towards the **sacrum** and the head, or diagonally, towards one shoulder and the opposite hip. At the end of the stretch, let your hands rest in an **energy balancing** hold.

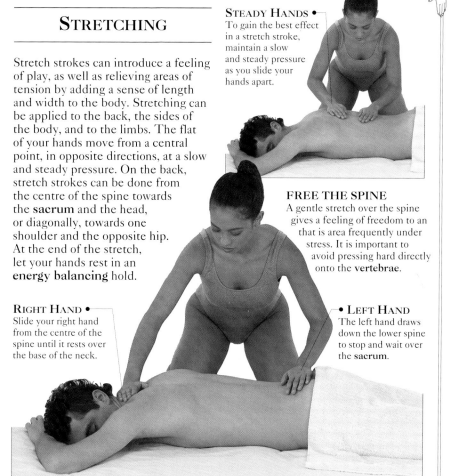

STEADY HANDS •
To gain the best effect in a stretch stroke, maintain a slow and steady pressure as you slide your hands apart.

FREE THE SPINE
A gentle stretch over the spine gives a feeling of freedom to an that is area frequently under stress. It is important to avoid pressing hard directly onto the **vertebrae**.

RIGHT HAND •
Slide your right hand from the centre of the spine until it rests over the base of the neck.

• LEFT HAND
The left hand draws down the lower spine to stop and wait over the **sacrum**.

FEATHERING

RELAX YOUR HANDS
Complete your effleurage strokes on the back with delicate feather touches, which will heighten the sensitivity of your partner's skin. Using just your fingertips, with the minimum of pressure, run one hand after the other down the whole surface of the back several times. Most people, except the ticklish, love the tingling effect of feathering, and it is a delightful way to finish a massage. Try varying the speed and pressure.

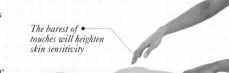
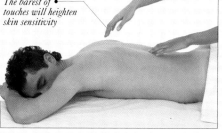

The barest of • touches will heighten skin sensitivity

SKILL

7 KNEADING

Definition: *Rolling and squeezing the flesh away from the bone*

KNEADING IS A DEEPER LEVEL of massage, once the muscles have warmed up and relaxed from soothing strokes, and the oil has soaked into the skin. The rolling and squeezing action is perfect for fleshy areas of the body such as the calves, thighs, and buttocks, bringing suppleness to the muscles, and helping to eliminate toxins, which can cause stiffness and pain, from the tissue. Always precede and follow up your kneading with effleurage, to soothe and harmonize your strokes. In this sequence, you will work on the legs.

OBJECTIVE: To bring invigoration to tired muscles. *Rating* •••••

PREPARING THE AREA

When you have completed the effleurage massage on the back, make a connection hold between the upper and lower body. Apply the oil by stroking it down the legs. Relax the whole leg, from ankle to pelvis, with long, soothing **main strokes**. Give a stretch to the leg with a gentle pull, as your hands glide firmly back. Follow up with other effleurage strokes, before applying kneading, first to the calf, then the thigh.

Bring your partner's awareness to his body

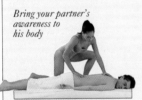

Apply oil to the legs before you begin effleurage

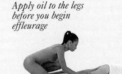

Relax the whole area with long, soothing **main strokes**

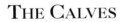

THE CALVES

For broad kneading, place your thumbs on the centre of the calf's muscle bulk, supporting the leg with your fingers. Using pressure from the heels and sides of the thumbs, make continuous alternate circular motions, moving upwards. When your hands are just below the knee, glide them back down to repeat, adding pressure.

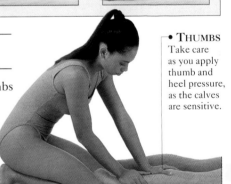

• THUMBS
Take care as you apply thumb and heel pressure, as the calves are sensitive.

THE THIGHS

Kneading will bring flexibility to the broad expanse of muscle in the thighs, enlivening it by boosting the blood supply and increasing the exchange of tissue fluids. After applying effleurage strokes, move to the opposite side of the body so that you can knead more effectively on the sides of the leg.

FIRST STAGE
Place both hands on the thigh, with fingers pointing away from yourself and thumbs at an angle. Applying pressure with one hand, scoop and squeeze the flesh between the thumb and fingers. Roll the tissue towards the other hand.

• ELBOWS
Holding your elbows at a slight angle from the body with your wrists loose and your hands supple, create an effect like kneading dough.

HANDS •
One hand alternates rhythmically with the other, pushing and squeezing the flesh back and forth in a rounded, wave-like motion.

SECOND STAGE
Push and release the flesh into the waiting hand, which in turn will gather it up and return it, so that the muscle tissue rolls to and fro continuously. Move up and down the thigh in strips.

THE BUTTOCKS

Tension often resides deep in the large **gluteal** muscles of the buttocks, caused by bad **posture**, a stiff back, or sexual and emotional stress. You may wish to massage the buttocks as a continuation of the work on the legs, or include them in the back massage.

WRINGING
Introduce a wringing effect to increase the squeeze on the muscle. With additional pressure, twist the flesh slightly as you roll it back and forth.

• SCOOP FLESH
Scoop the flesh towards the thumb, as you knead the whole area thoroughly, reaching around the sides by the hips and pelvis.

SKILL

7

THE BACK

Now that you have learnt invigorating kneading on the legs and buttocks, you can experiment with these revitalizing movements to the back. When combined with relaxing effleurage strokes, you will be giving a substantial massage that targets key tension areas of the body: around the shoulder blades, over the shoulders, and at the base of the neck. Begin by following the whole sequence of effleurage strokes on the back (see pp.38-39 and 46-49), ensuring one movement flows into the next.

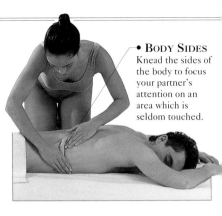

• BODY SIDES
Knead the sides of the body to focus your partner's attention on an area which is seldom touched.

KNEADING ALONG THE BODY
Knead along your partner's sides from the hips and waistline, towards the shoulder blades. If there is too little flesh to lift from the ribs, soften your touch to massage more lightly.

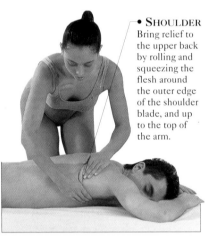

• SHOULDER
Bring relief to the upper back by rolling and squeezing the flesh around the outer edge of the shoulder blade, and up to the top of the arm.

THE SHOULDERS

Almost everyone experiences pain or stiffness in their shoulders at some time. This is often due to our **posture** in standing, sitting, and movement. Hunching over a desk, or bracing and raising our shoulders unconsciously in stress, all add to our discomfort, as do tiredness, fear, and anger. Your partner will enjoy the revitalizing effects of this stroke as it loosens the muscles, frees stiffness, shifts tension, and allows the blood to circulate more freely towards the head.

KNEADING THE UPPER BACK
Above: Kneading brings greater flexibility to the network of muscles that runs above and beneath the shoulder blades.

KNEADING A TIGHT SPOT
Right: Knead across the top of the shoulder on the opposite side from you, modifying your strokes to reach and penetrate the narrow area between the top of the shoulder blade and the base of the neck.

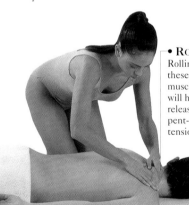

• ROLL
Rolling these muscles will help release pent-up tension.

BOTH SHOULDERS

To knead both shoulders at once, hook your fingers lightly over the shoulders to anchor your hands. Scoop the flesh upwards with your heels and thumbs, squeezing and releasing it gently. Knead well into both shoulders until you feel the muscles responding, and follow up with effleurage. Cross to the opposite side and repeat the whole kneading sequence shown on these pages. Cover the surface of the back with long soft strokes to integrate your kneading into the massage, and finish with an **energy balancing** hold.

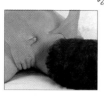

NECK RELEASE
This stroke can release painful tension, often trapped between the base of the neck, and around the top of the shoulder blades.

SHOULDERS •
The benefits of having relaxed shoulders are immediately obvious. Not only does it increase physical comfort, it also reduces mental anxiety.

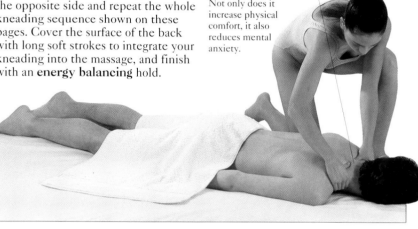

APPLYING KNEADING

FRONT OF THE BODY
The front of the body is generally more sensitive and vulnerable, so there are fewer areas where you can apply deep strokes. Knead to relax and invigorate wherever flesh amply covers the bones, after soothing with soft strokes.

THE LIMBS
On the legs, knead the fleshy areas alongside the shin bone, the knee, and then work thoroughly over the thigh. You may need to adapt your kneading strokes to the narrow shape of the arm, see below. Try supporting the underarm with your fingers, and work both hands up over the muscles in a flowing sequence of alternate circular motions. Squeeze the flesh as your heels and thumbs apply pressure on the outward half-circle. Return the stroke more lightly. This action releases muscular tension as it rolls tissue from the bone.

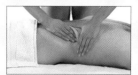

ABDOMEN
Knead and wring the **external oblique muscles** of the abdominal area.

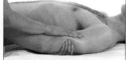

ARMS
Gently squeeze the **biceps** and **triceps**, during your circular kneading strokes.

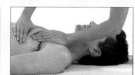

PECTORALS
The **pectorals** in the upper chest respond well to kneading (see also p.66).

8 PETRISSAGE

Definition: *Strokes which push the tissue towards the bone*

PETRISSAGE IS APPLIED with fingertips, thumb pads, heels, or knuckles, which are sunk into **soft tissue** at a steady pressure, to stretch and manipulate. It is particularly useful for working into tissue surrounding bone – alongside the spine, the shin, the knee, the elbow, under the skull, and around the shoulder blades. Petrissage can be applied whenever toxins and trapped waste products are felt as small nodules or granular deposits in the tissue. The stroke grinds tissue against bone, and disperses toxins into the **circulatory system**, for elimination from the body. Never apply petrissage too fast, or too deep, or your partner will tense up. Sink into the tissue slowly, allowing it to yield to your pressure gradually.

OBJECTIVE: To release deep tension, and eliminate toxins. *Rating* •••••

–STROKES SEQUENCE –

Because **petrissage** uses an increased level of pressure, it is important that muscles are warm and relaxed first through effleurage and kneading. This skill shows how to apply petrissage to the front of the leg, in the following sequence: after applying oil, begin with three main effleurage strokes to the whole leg, follow up with soft strokes, and kneading of the shin and knee area. Apply deeper petrissage movements up alongside the shin and around the kneecap. Integrate strokes over whole leg with a long stroke, and then relax the thigh with effleurage, kneading, and petrissage. Complete with **main strokes**, feathering, and connection holds, and repeat the sequence on the other leg.

PREPARATION

Effleurage strokes relax the leg and boost circulation, as kneading warms and invigorates the leg muscles.

THE LOWER LEG

The lower leg bears a large proportion of body weight, and is supported by the shin bone, or tibia, and a thinner bone, the fibula, which run parallel from knee to ankle. A deep **petrissage** stroke between these bones, from the ankle area slowly up to the knee joint, helps release strain from this area.

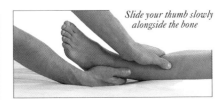

Slide your thumb slowly alongside the bone

SHIN STROKE

Pull gently on the heel to give slight traction in the leg, and sink your other thumb pad into the channel running along the outer edge of the tibia. Slide slowly upwards to the knee. Glide your hand back to repeat three times.

THE KNEE

The mobility of the knee is vital in support and locomotion of the body. **Petrissage** helps to relax the **ligaments** and **tendons** that bind the bones and muscles together. Three long bones meet at the knee joint – the femur of the thigh, and the tibia and fibula of the lower leg. The patella, or kneecap, protects the front of the knee joint.

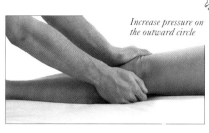

Increase pressure on the outward circle

USE YOUR HEELS ON THE KNEE
Support the back of the knee joint with your fingers. Use your heels to apply pressure, by rotating hands alternately over each side.

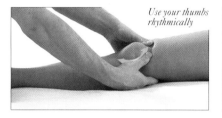

Use your thumbs rhythmically

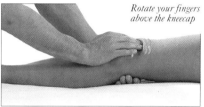

Rotate your fingers above the kneecap

ENCIRCLING THE KNEECAP
Glide your thumbs from the top to the base of the kneecap so that they slightly overlap, and then back up again. Repeat several times.

USING YOUR FINGERTIPS
Clasp behind the knee firmly with one hand, and use the fingertips of your other hand to make tiny circles around the top of the knee.

THE THIGH

The muscles of the thigh are bulky as they must support the body's weight and movement. Beneath the muscles is the largest bone in the body, the femur. These two **petrissage** strokes will aid release of muscular tension.

PRESSURE
Move up over the thigh with firm, alternate fan strokes, using your heels to add pressure.

THIGH MUSCLES
Sink the heel of one hand into the area just above the knee, and slowly slide it upwards.

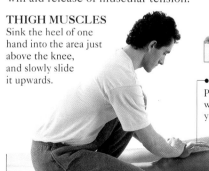

• INCREASE YOUR PRESSURE
Place your other hand across your wrist for increased pressure. Lighten your stroke at the top of the thigh.

SKILL
8

PETRISSAGE ON SPINE

*Applying **petrissage** strokes to relax the **sacrum** and **vertebral column***

WORKING ON THE SPINE

Having practised **petrissage** on the front of the leg, you can now apply it to those areas of the body you have already massaged. Use petrissage in conjunction with your other strokes, such as effleurage and kneading, so the tissue is well prepared. The back is an area which responds particularly well to petrissage, so use it to supplement your strokes, soothing the **sacrum** and relaxing the lower back. Releasing tension from alongside the spine will bring increased flexibility to the long muscles that support the **vertebrae**, and improve the body's **posture**.

SACRUM

The **sacrum** is the flat, triangular bone at the base of the spine, which also forms part of the pelvic girdle. Massage, on and around the sacrum, can feel extremely comforting and will help to release the stress imposed on the lower spine, by harmful **postural** habits or muscular strain.

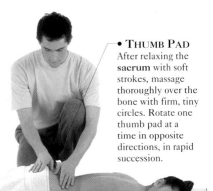

• THUMB PAD
After relaxing the **sacrum** with soft strokes, massage thoroughly over the bone with firm, tiny circles. Rotate one thumb pad at a time in opposite directions, in rapid succession.

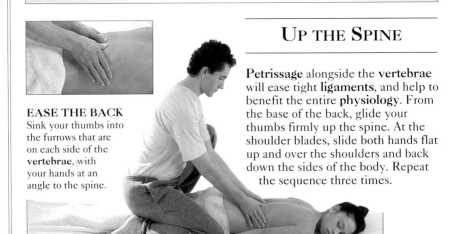

EASE THE BACK
Sink your thumbs into the furrows that are on each side of the **vertebrae**, with your hands at an angle to the spine.

UP THE SPINE

Petrissage alongside the **vertebrae** will ease tight **ligaments**, and help to benefit the entire **physiology**. From the base of the back, glide your thumbs firmly up the spine. At the shoulder blades, slide both hands flat up and over the shoulders and back down the sides of the body. Repeat the sequence three times.

DOWN THE BACK

When massaging from this position behind your partner's head, use **petrissage** from top to bottom, by applying pressure with your thumbs simultaneously down each side of the spinal column. Place your hands at a slight angle to each other and flat on the surface of the back, and work down as far as you can reach in comfort. Sweep up around the sides of the body and over the shoulders to repeat the stroke twice. Follow up with the thumb roll stroke (see inset) alongside the spine from top to bottom, one side after the other.

THUMB ROLL
Slide your thumbs down alongside the spine. Repeatedly roll the leading thumb back over the other one.

• THUMBS
Work your thumbs over areas wherever you can feel sore, hard, and knotted spots, to dissolve tension and toxins.

OTHER PETRISSAGE

Adapt **petrissage** to suit any particular area of the body, especially wherever tension gathers in tissue over and around bone. Learn to apply the optimum pressure from different parts of your hands, to achieve relief of tight, sore spots. Check with your partner to see if you are applying a satisfying level of pressure and speed.

DON'T PUSH TOO HARD
Never penetrate a muscle area too quickly, or push against resistance, as the body will contract further in defence. The art of a successful petrissage stroke is to sink pressure into the tissue only as far as it is willing to yield, and to take enough time to allow the area to relax. It takes practice to achieve the correct application of these deeper pressure strokes. As you learn the other massage skills in this course, and use them around the body, you will find that petrissage, when used in conjunction with your other strokes, deepens and enhances the total relaxation of your partner.

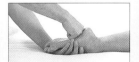

FOOT
During a foot massage, you can use the flat edge of your knuckles to create a firm stretch over the sole.

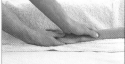

ARM
Gliding your thumb pad slowly up between the two long bones of the forearm will ease away tension.

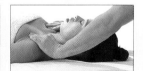

COLLAR BONE
While massaging the chest, slide your forefinger and thumb along the area either side of the collar bone.

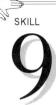

SKILL

9 PERCUSSION

Definition: *Vibratory movements performed on fleshy areas*

PERCUSSION IS A SERIES OF RAPID MOVEMENTS on the surface of the skin. Their best use is as a stimulating conclusion to your massage, to bring a feeling of life to your partner. However, if the intention of your massage is to be wholly relaxing, or if your partner has fallen asleep, omit them. The three strokes described here are cupping, hacking, and pummelling. Their brisk action brings tone to muscle tissue, stimulates nerve endings, and draws the blood supply up to the skin, to leave the body warm and glowing. They are excellent when following up after kneading and **petrissage**. Apply percussion only over fleshy, muscular areas, avoiding bones and varicose veins.

OBJECTIVE: To stimulate, invigorate, and bring tone to muscle tissue during massage. *Rating* •••

CUPPING

Bend your palms at the knuckles, with your fingers straight and your thumbs drawn inwards. This creates a vacuum in the centre of your hands during rapid cupping, so that the blood is drawn towards the surface of the skin.

DRUMMING
Lightly drum the calf muscles, one cupped hand following the other in quick succession, so the strokes flick back off the skin.

HANDS •
Your hands should make a sound like the beat of horses' hooves as cupping expels the air rapidly from under your hands.

ALTERNATE
Cupping the fleshy area of the thighs helps to improve muscle tone, and increase toxin elimination.

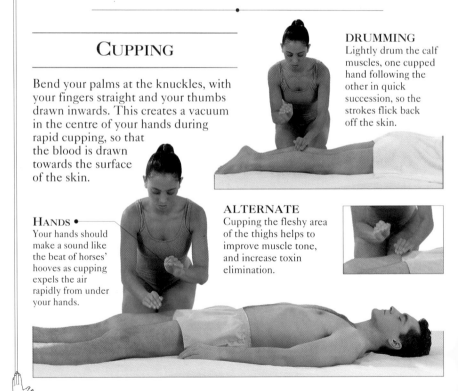

SOFT FISTS
Soft fists create the right effect for pummelling on fleshy areas.

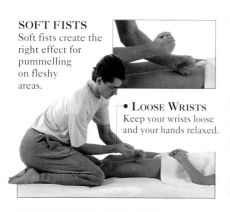

• LOOSE WRISTS
Keep your wrists loose and your hands relaxed.

PUMMELLING

Pummelling uses the loose fists of both hands to drum on muscular areas such as the thighs and buttocks, to loosen and invigorate underlying tissue. As with other **percussion** strokes, let your hands spring back off the skin, one after the other, to gain maximum effect. This will produce a gentle, but vigorous pummelling, which stimulates the whole area.

• BOUNCE
The success of hacking is in letting your hands bounce off the skin.

HACKING

Keep your shoulders, wrists, and hands relaxed, so that the hacking strokes do not feel like karate chops. Use the sides of your hands alternately to strike rapidly on shoulders, buttocks, and backs of legs. Avoid striking directly onto bone, bruising, or broken veins.

SHOULDERS
The sides of your hands can work into the often tense, narrow areas of muscle around the shoulders.

• RHYTHMIC HANDS
Use your hands rhythmically as if playing a drum, to avoid the effect becoming monotonous or heavy.

TAPOTEMENT

Tapotement is a fast, vibratory movement made by shaking an area of muscle with the end of the fingertips of one, or both hands. It is a stimulatory motion which helps to loosen up tight areas.

Tapotement is generally used on small muscles, such as in the cheeks of the face, but it can be an effective way of shaking and loosening muscle on larger areas, such as the thighs and buttocks.

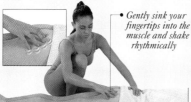

• Gently sink your fingertips into the muscle and shake rhythmically

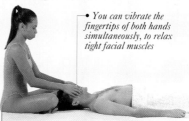

• You can vibrate the fingertips of both hands simultaneously, to relax tight facial muscles

10 MASSAGE FOR STRESS RELIEF

Definition: *A face, head, and neck massage designed for relief from stress and tension*

STRESS IS A COMMON PROBLEM in the modern world. This massage sequence brings relaxation to the face, head, and neck, by focusing on key areas where tension accumulates as a result of anxiety, emotions, and physical stress. It can be used as a short massage in itself, or combined in a full body session. From a position above your partner's head, begin with an **energy balancing** hold, placing your hands symmetrically around the crown of the head. Ease tension from the neck and under the skull, by lifting and rolling the head, as described in the Passive Movements on page 34.

OBJECTIVE: A short massage that relaxes and calms the whole body by helping to alleviate stress symptoms. *Rating* •••••

THE BROWS

Place your thumb pads just under the brow bone

Rest your hands softly around your partner's head, with your thumbs on the centre of the brow just above the eyebrows. Glide your thumbs steadily outwards, and complete with a rounded sweep of the temples. The temples are delicate areas that respond wonderfully to massage. Progress the stroke up the brow to massage the whole area.

TEMPLE SWEEP •
Lighten your stroke as your circular sweep around the temples turns back in towards the face. Always withdraw your thumbs slowly from the contact.

EYEBROWS
Above: Make a firm slide of the thumb pads from the inner to outer corners of the eyebrows. Finish with a sweep of the temples.

THE EYES

Softly stroking all around the eyes with your fingertips, from the inner edge to the outer edge, can soothe away tiredness and stress. Never press hard on this sensitive area or drag on the soft skin. If your partner wears contact lenses, ask her to remove them before the massage.

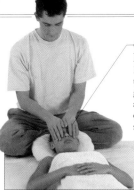

• WARM HANDS
Rub your hands together to generate heat, and place them over the eyes for several moments.

Left: Make firm petrissage strokes around the cheeks

THE CHEEKS

People often unconsciously tighten their facial muscles when suppressing their feelings, which leads to a tight, mask-like effect, particularly around the cheeks and mouth. Firm **petrissage** strokes, far left, will begin to alleviate this. Glide your thumb pads down the sides of the nose into the muscle below the cheek bone, drawing out to the sides of the head. Then sweep your hands through the hair, and return to repeat this stroke twice more.

LOOSEN CHEEKS
Right: Sink your fingertips into the fleshy cheeks, and rotate them several times, one area at a time.

THE JAW

Some of the strongest muscles of the body are in the jaw. Kneading and stroking relaxes these muscles. Place your index fingers beneath the chin and knead over it with short, alternating strokes from your thumbs. As the chin and jaw relax, the whole face softens.

KNEAD CHIN •
Moving your fingers and thumbs, knead up over one side of the jawbone and then the other.

STROKE JAW
Alternating hands, tenderly stroke along the jaw line.

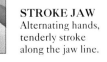

SKILL

10 THE EARS

Your partner will love this ear massage which has a delightfully relaxing effect on the whole body. Work simultaneously over both ears, making tiny circular movements with your forefingers, and squeezing gently against your thumbs. Stroke in the folds behind the ears with your middle fingers.

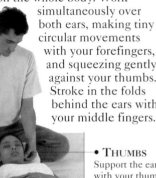

• THUMBS
Support the ear with your thumb, while you rub gently with your fingertips.

— CONNECTION HOLD —

Now that you have massaged the face, you are ready to work on the neck. Start with a relaxing connection hold, placing your right hand gently across the forehead, while the left hand supports the back of the neck, with fingers pointing in opposite directions. Wait a few moments until you feel the neck area relaxing into your hand.

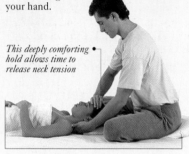

This deeply comforting hold allows time to release neck tension

SHOULDERS TO NECK

The base of the neck tightens under stress, often reducing the circulation of blood to the brain, which can cause tension headaches. To manipulate taut neck muscles, place one hand beneath the base of the neck. Gently squeeze the muscles while pulling your hand upwards. Release your hold as your other hand repeats the action.

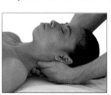

MILKING STROKE
Alternate your hands so there is continuous motion between both hands. This important stroke on the neck muscles needs some practice to achieve its milking effect.

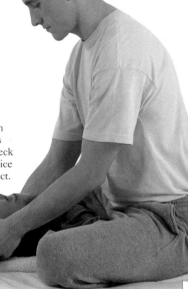

THE NECK

Roll your partner's head to one side and support it in one hand. Place your other hand at an angle below the skull and slide firmly down the exposed side of the neck, adding pressure with your heel, to stretch the **trapezius muscle**. Soften the pressure and flex your wrist, as your hand sweeps around the shoulder joint, and glides up behind the neck and out of the head and hair. Repeat this stroke three times in a flowing sequence.

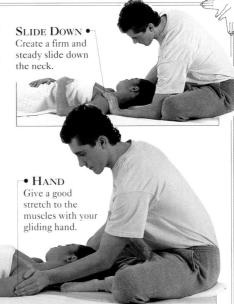

SLIDE DOWN •
Create a firm and steady slide down the neck.

• HAND
Give a good stretch to the muscles with your gliding hand.

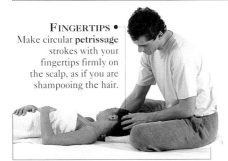

FINGERTIPS •
Make circular **petrissage** strokes with your fingertips firmly on the scalp, as if you are shampooing the hair.

THE SCALP

Massaging the scalp helps to loosen the thin layer of muscle covering the skull, which feels very refreshing. Make small, brisk circles with your fingertips, from the base of the skull to the crown. Now apply all the neck and scalp strokes on the other side.

FINISHING STROKES

When you have completed all the strokes in this stress-relief massage, and your partner is feeling relaxed, bring the head in line with the spine, ready for a finishing stroke. Slide your hands under the shoulders to rest, palms upward, each side of the spine. Bring deeper release and extension to the neck muscles by slowly drawing your hands upwards and outwards behind the head, taking care to lift it slightly as your hands pass under the hairline. Now pull your fingers gently through the hair to create an hypnotic and soothing finish. This brings the stress-relief massage to a relaxing close, which has helped to ease tension from the face, neck, head, and scalp.

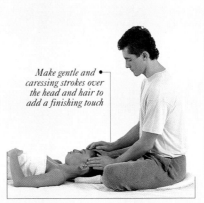

Make gentle and caressing strokes over the head and hair to add a finishing touch

SKILL

11

DAY 2

SENSITIVE AREAS

Definition: *Massage on the chest and abdominal areas of the body*

THE MORE YOU MASSAGE, the greater the feeling that whenever you touch a person's body, you are also evoking change within the mind and emotions. This is the **holistic** principle of massage – that the whole person is affected by massage, and not just the physical body, and so the body should always be approached with a high degree of respect. The chest and abdominal areas of the body not only protect vital organs, but also hold powerful emotions within the muscle structure. Working on the front of the body, you will immediately feel that you are making contact with more emotional aspects of your partner. Massage allows your partner to assimilate those emotions, along with the release of tension in a gentle and safe way, as breathing increases and muscles relax beneath your strokes.

OBJECTIVE: Strokes to aid physical and emotional relaxation. *Rating* •••••

THE CHEST

*The **thoracic cavity** contains the heart and lungs, protected by the structure of the ribcage. Your massage should help relaxation, and full, vital breathing*

CONNECTION HOLD

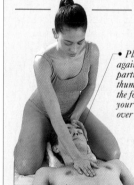

• *Place your left hand against the side of your partner's head with the thumb resting softly on the forehead. Bring your right hand to rest over the heart area*

Apply your strokes to the chest after the face and neck massage (see pp.60-63). To integrate both areas of the body, begin with a connection hold. This will have a sedative effect on your partner, giving him time to relax and to bring his awareness to the emotionally vulnerable heart area, and to breathe more fully. The warm touch of your hands will be reassuring, and enable your partner to connect more deeply with any underlying feelings, which can surface and be released gently. Close your eyes, and become aware of your **breath flow**, with your touch light yet vital.

THE RIBCAGE

The flowing and repetitive sweep of an effleurage **main stroke** (see p.45) over the surface of the ribcage, across the **pectoral** muscles, and up behind the shoulders and neck, will immediately begin to relieve constriction of the **thoracic** region, and increase lung capacity. This improves the delivery of oxygen and nutrients to cells throughout the body. Repeat the main stroke at least three times, varying your pressure, and fully encompassing the contours of the upper body.

FANNING •
These strokes will warm the ribcage. Apply pressure on the down and outward motion, returning to the source of the stroke more lightly.

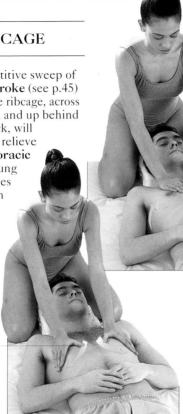

• WRISTS
Swivel your wrists to glide your palms smoothly out towards the shoulders, when your hands return to the chest from the sides of the ribcage.

MAIN STROKE
Above: After completing the stroke, pull up behind the neck and head, to sweep tension right away.

FAN STROKES
Left: Follow up the **main stroke** by fanning down the ribcage. Repeat the fan sequence three times.

• PRESS SHOULDERS
Press down on the shoulders with your palms, to expand the upper chest. The top of the lungs extend as far up as the shoulders, which should start rising with increased inhalation.

THE SHOULDERS

Shoulders act as protective armour to the body, shielding it from stress or painful feelings. They tend to stiffen, brace, or hunch forward in situations of pressure. All this can cause the muscles of the chest and back to overextend or contract, affecting a person's wellbeing. Breathing is diminished and **posture** becomes unbalanced. Help to loosen up and expand the upper chest by applying your own weight down through your hands, onto both shoulders, with a steady pressure. The shoulders will open and drop back towards the mattress. Hold for several moments before releasing the pressure slowly.

SKILL

11

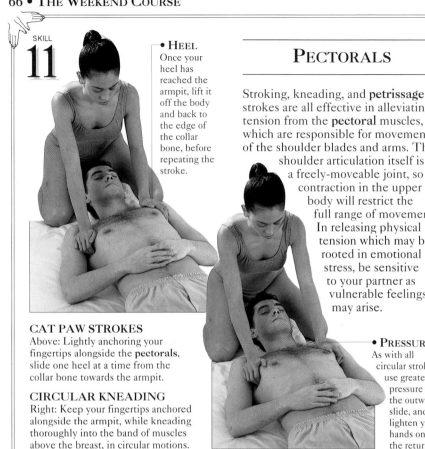

• HEEL
Once your heel has reached the armpit, lift it off the body and back to the edge of the collar bone, before repeating the stroke.

PECTORALS

Stroking, kneading, and **petrissage** strokes are all effective in alleviating tension from the **pectoral** muscles, which are responsible for movement of the shoulder blades and arms. The shoulder articulation itself is a freely-moveable joint, so contraction in the upper body will restrict the full range of movement. In releasing physical tension which may be rooted in emotional stress, be sensitive to your partner as vulnerable feelings may arise.

• PRESSURE
As with all circular strokes, use greater pressure on the outward slide, and lighten your hands on the return.

CAT PAW STROKES
Above: Lightly anchoring your fingertips alongside the **pectorals**, slide one heel at a time from the collar bone towards the armpit.

CIRCULAR KNEADING
Right: Keep your fingertips anchored alongside the armpit, while kneading thoroughly into the band of muscles above the breast, in circular motions.

SPREADING HANDS
Finish the chest massage with flowing **main strokes**, adding extra pressure with your heels as they diverge over the **pectorals**.

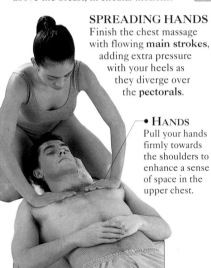

• HANDS
Pull your hands firmly towards the shoulders to enhance a sense of space in the upper chest.

——— CONNECTION ———

Move to kneel at your partner's side, and make a connection hold over the heart and abdominal area. Let your hands impart a feeling of harmony between the upper and lower half of the torso. The chest and abdomen are separated by the large diaphragm muscle, which often becomes constricted under stress. Allow your touch to encourage connection, relaxation, and deeper breathing.

This "laying of hands" will bring a sense of wholeness to your partner

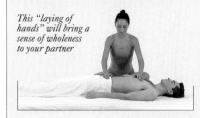

THE BELLY

Strokes to use on the sensitive area of the belly, to ease away nervous tension,
aid digestion, and increase emotional relaxation

CIRCULAR STROKES

Many people find it difficult to allow
anyone to touch their belly because
it feels so sensitive and defenceless.
Once the area relaxes, however, it
can be wonderfully comforting to
have it stroked. Always approach the
abdominal area slowly and carefully.

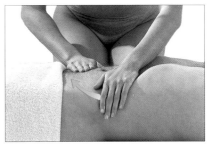

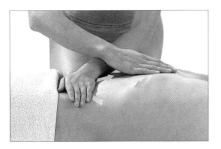

DECREASING THE CIRCLES
Above: Melt away tension with large circular
strokes in a clockwise direction (see p.42),
then spiralling inwards to focus on the centre
of the belly, before taking them out again.

THE HALF-CIRCLE
Left: Lift one hand to allow the leading hand
to complete the full circle. The hand returns
to the body to emphasize the last half-circle.
These strokes give a lovely hypnotic effect.

• **CO-ORDINATION**
Make clockwise and
anti-clockwise circles
simultaneously with
your hands. This
stroke will need some
practice before you
feel confident in
achieving its flowing
figure-of-eight shape.

FIGURE-OF-EIGHT

This is a great stroke for relaxing the
lower abdomen and sides. Place your
hands, fingers pointing away, over
each side of the body. Slide hands
diagonally past each other to
encircle the sides of the
body, before gliding back
again to curve around
the opposite side.

• **FLOWING STROKE**
Take the stroke in a
continuous unbroken
flow, up and down over
the torso several times.

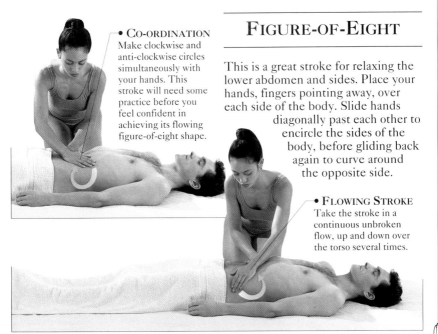

SKILL

11

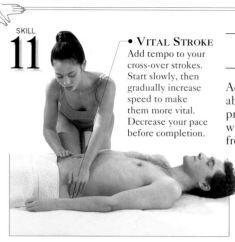

• **VITAL STROKE**
Add tempo to your
cross-over strokes.
Start slowly, then
gradually increase
speed to make
them more vital.
Decrease your pace
before completion.

CROSS-OVER

Adapt these familiar strokes to the
abdominal area, to complement the
previous strokes to the belly. Start
with cross-over strokes working up
from hips to ribcage and back down
again. Place your hands, fingers
pointing away, on each side of the
body, and begin to slide hands
continuously past each other,
moving up the body. Make sure
your hands reach right down to
the mattress on both sides.

MILKING STROKES

Massage should accentuate the
sensual, sculptural shape of the body,
and milking strokes (see p.48) along
the sides of the torso are perfect for
this. Slide your hands, one after the
other, from under the body, over the
side, towards the centre of the belly.

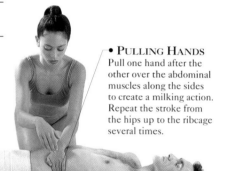

• **PULLING HANDS**
Pull one hand after the
other over the abdominal
muscles along the sides
to create a milking action.
Repeat the stroke from
the hips up to the ribcage
several times.

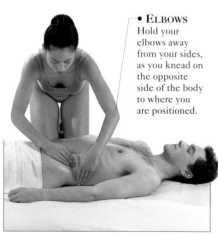

• **ELBOWS**
Hold your
elbows away
from your sides,
as you knead on
the opposite
side of the body
to where you
are positioned.

KNEADING

Kneading will loosen and invigorate
the muscles that wrap around the
body, from the belly to the spine.
These muscles give support to the
abdominal organs and the **vertebral
column**, and their strength and
flexibility are essential for comfort
and good **posture**. Knead the flesh
with both hands, up and down from
the pelvic girdle to the ribcage.
When you have finished, repeat the
sequence of strokes on this page on
the other side of your partner's body.

DIAPHRAGM

The diaphragm is a large dome-shaped muscle that attaches to the ribcage at the front, and to the lower **vertebrae** at the back of the body. It is central to the breathing process, as the contraction and relaxation of the diaphragm decrease and increase the air pressure in the lungs, to facilitate inspiration and expiration. The diaphragm is too deep within the body to be reached by **soft tissue** massage, but relaxation of the area surrounding the ribcage will help to relieve overall tension, and improve breathing.

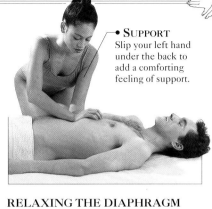

• SUPPORT
Slip your left hand under the back to add a comforting feeling of support.

RELAXING THE DIAPHRAGM
Above: Keep your right hand relaxed and raised slightly off the body, while using its heel to massage in circular motions below the ribcage, and around the diaphragm area.

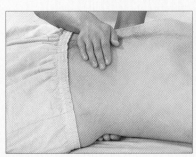

• CONNECT
Connect the areas above and below the diaphragm with a sweeping effleurage stroke.

EFFLEURAGE

From the base of the breastbone, fan your hands upwards and outwards to the sides of the body. Slide your fingers under the back while gliding your hands firmly down to the hip area. Encircle the pelvic girdle, and then swivel your wrists so that your hands stroke back up to the base of the sternum. Repeat this stroke three times without a break.

HOLDING YOUR PARTNER

Now give your partner time to connect with and assimilate any feelings that may have arisen, as muscular tension dissolves and breathing deepens. Cradle your partner's abdomen and back between your hands to give him a feeling of support, on both a physical and emotional level. These periods of stillness in massage directly affect the **autonomic nervous system**, enabling it to restore balance and rest to overstressed organs and equilibrium to the mind. Slide one hand beneath the lower back, and as it relaxes downwards place your other hand over the belly. Channel your own **breath flow** into your hands, and hold for as long as feels appropriate.

This supportive hold relaxes the belly to bring warmth and increased oxygen to vital organs

SKILL

DAY 2

12 LIMBS

Definition: *Techniques for the arms, hands, legs, and feet*

WHEN YOU LEARN HOW to implement the right strokes on the body's limbs and extremities, your partner's awareness of their body as a connected unity will increase. This adds to the sense of physical and emotional integration. The **postural** structure of a person's arms and hands often reflects their attitudes to creativity and outward communication. The legs and feet, which are the body's foundation, indicate the inner relationship with stability and movement.

OBJECTIVE: To increase flexibility and body balance. *Rating* •••••

ARMS

Strokes to release tension from the muscles and joints of the arms

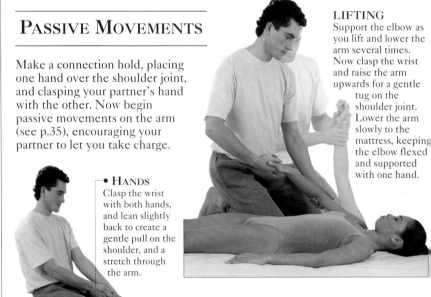

PASSIVE MOVEMENTS

Make a connection hold, placing one hand over the shoulder joint, and clasping your partner's hand with the other. Now begin passive movements on the arm (see p.35), encouraging your partner to let you take charge.

LIFTING
Support the elbow as you lift and lower the arm several times. Now clasp the wrist and raise the arm upwards for a gentle tug on the shoulder joint. Lower the arm slowly to the mattress, keeping the elbow flexed and supported with one hand.

• HANDS
Clasp the wrist with both hands, and lean slightly back to create a gentle pull on the shoulder, and a stretch through the arm.

STRETCHING
Left: An easy stretch helps to release tension from contracted muscles surrounding the "ball-and-socket" shoulder joints. Slowly release the taut arm back into a relaxed position.

FLEXING THE WRISTS

There are eight small carpal bones in each wrist, and the intercarpal joints are known as "gliding" joints. Pain or stiffness can result from repetitive movement or **postural** stress, which may tighten **ligaments** and affect the hand's mobility. To aid suppleness, flex and extend the wrist, and rotate the hand several times.

ROTATING WRIST
Rotate the hand three times to the left and right. Try to gain maximum movement without overexerting the natural motion of the joint.

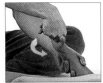

SUPPORT
Clasp your partner's arm just above the wrist, as a support. Take hold of her hand, to enable you to move the wrist.

• FLEX THE WRIST
Exercise the gliding joints and **ligaments** by carefully flexing and extending the wrist as you gently bend the hand back and forth.

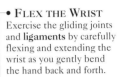

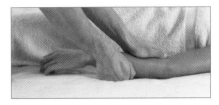

THE ARM MASSAGE

After passive movements, relax the arm by applying a **main stroke** three times. Incorporate the strokes shown right and below, into your effleurage, kneading, and **petrissage** sequence on the lower and upper arm, adapting your strokes to the arm's narrow shape. Integrate all your strokes with flowing effleurage before massaging the hand.

RELAXING THE FOREARM
Make a series of small, rounded fan strokes, from wrist to elbow, one hand following the other. Slide your hands gently back to the wrist, and repeat the sequence three times.

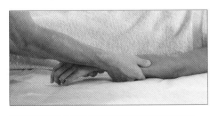

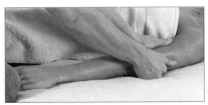

PETRISSAGE BETWEEN BONES
Take the hand into your own, and slightly raise the forearm. Place your thumb pad between the **radius** and **ulna** bones at the wrist, and slide firmly upward to the elbow.

STRETCHING UPPER ARM
Support the underside of the upper arm with your fingers, while sliding your thumbs and heels outwards to create a transverse stretch across the muscle bulk. Repeat several times.

HANDS

*These strokes bring relaxation and suppleness to the hands, and
can precede or follow an arm massage*

THE HAND MASSAGE

Hands are usually so active, that they
seldom have the chance simply to
receive touch. This is why a hand
massage can feel so surprisingly
enjoyable and calming.

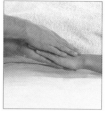

HOLDING
Lay your partner's
hand between your
own and hold it
gently. Let the
warmth of your
hands melt away
tension, giving your
partner time to relax.

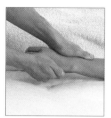

MAKE SUPPLE
Supporting the palm
with your fingers,
use your heels and
thumbs to stroke in
alternate circles,
from the knuckles to
the wrist. Glide back
down, and repeat.

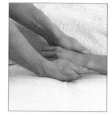

STRETCHING
Stretch the top of
the hand by sliding
your thumbs and
heels firmly across
to its edges. Support
the palm with
your fingers, as you
repeat several times.

PULL FINGERS
Pull firmly along the
top and bottom of
each finger, with
your thumb and
index finger. Work
from base to tip,
giving an extra
squeeze to the tip.

PULL THUMBS
Swop hands so you
can pull along the
thumb. Massage the
base of the thumb
and the fleshy web
by the forefinger,
with your fingertips,
heel, and thumb.

TENDONS
Hold the hand in your
own, and use your
other thumb to stroke
steadily up between
the **tendons** on the
back of the hand. Sink
your thumb into the
channels between
the tendons, from
knuckles to wrist.

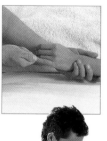

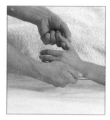

HAND ANATOMY

There are twenty seven bones in each
hand. These are activated by muscles
attached to the **humerus** bone in the
upper arm, and the **ulna** and **radius**
bones in the forearm. Their **tendons**
insert into the hand bones, and create
a range of movement in the palm and
fingers. Thousands of nerve endings
in the palm and fingertips, add to our
highly developed tactile sense.
Massaging the hand increases
its dexterity, and stimulates
the nervous system, especially
when combined with strokes
applied to the arm.

INTERLOCK

Interlock your fingers with your partner's, so that only the middle finger is free.

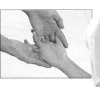

SMALL CIRCLES •
Use thumb pads to make continuous, alternate circles, fanning outwards.

THE PALM

Release muscular contraction, from the palm by pressing your fingers into the back of the hand. Massage the palm with your thumbs.

WRIST RELAXATION

A thick band of fibrous tissue binds the **tendons** close to the bones at the wrist, so any stiffness here will decrease the flexibility of the hand. Relax the wrist by stroking around both sides with your thumbs in small, alternate circles.

CONNECT

Support the hand, and continue the palm massage up to the soft skin of the wrist.

• **SUPPORT THE HAND**
Support the hand or forearm as you work on it, so that your partner can relax completely. Keep the elbow flexed on the mattress, to prevent the weight of the arm straining the joints.

INTEGRATING THE ARM STROKES

It is time to return your attention to the arm, to integrate your strokes on this limb. Start with soothing effleurage **main strokes**, sweeping up towards the shoulder. These will boost the **circulatory systems**, towards the heart and **lymph** glands. As your hands glide back down the arm, carry the stroke right out of your partner's hand. Feather lightly down the arm with delicate brushes of your fingertips, one hand following the other. Complete with an **energy balancing** hold, taking your partner's hand in your own, while placing your other hand gently over the heart area, for a restful finish. Repeat your strokes on the other arm and hand.

• *Feather lightly down the arm, from the shoulder towards the hand*

LEGS AND FEET

These massage strokes will help to relax the feet, ankles, and legs

—— CONNECTION ——

CONNECT BOTH FEET

Position yourself below your partner's feet. Sit on a small cushion so that your own **posture** remains comfortable. Begin the massage with a connection hold, placing your hands on top of the feet. This brings a sense of balance to the left and right sides of the body.

Calm your partner by • holding his feet for a while

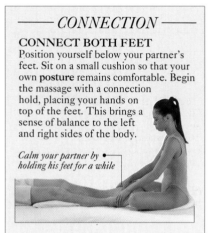

CRADLE FOOT

Start working on one foot by cradling it between your hands, focusing your whole attention and breath into your touch.

THE FEET

Feet are a masterpiece of anatomical design. A complex network of bones and muscles, forming three arches, can bear the body's weight in standing, and provide leverage in locomotion. A foot massage relaxes **postural** tension, and benefits the entire **physiological** system of the body, by the stimulation of the thousands of nerve endings that are located in the sole.

SIMPLE TOUCH •
Sometimes the simplest touch or hold can have profound effects. This foot hold draws energy away from an overactive mind down the body, to produce a sedative effect.

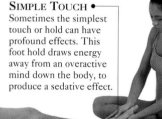

STROKE UP •
Rest your hands in opposite directions, little fingers leading, and stroke up from the toes to the ankle.

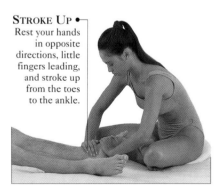

RELAX THE FOOT

Relax and warm the whole foot by stroking from toe to ankle. Fan your hands out around the ankle bones, gliding your fingers back along the sole. Repeat several times.

PRESSURE •
Press your fingers firmly into the sole of the foot. Increase the pressure on the outward fan movement of the circle, returning lightly to the source of your stroke each time.

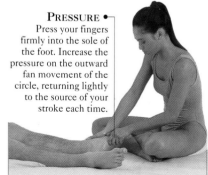

FAN STROKES

Supporting the foot with your fingers, fan the heels and thumbs of both hands in circular motions alternately, up over the instep to the the ankle. Glide hands back and repeat.

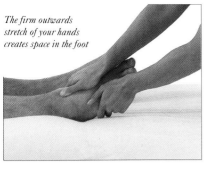

The firm outwards stretch of your hands creates space in the foot

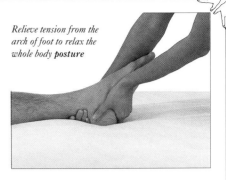

Relieve tension from the arch of foot to relax the whole body **posture**

SPREADING THE FOOT
The foot's intricate structure greatly benefits from this stretch. Press your fingers against the sole, and slide your heels and thumbs out towards the edges, working up to the ankle.

THE SOLE AND INSTEP
The smooth, broad surface of the heel of your hand fits perfectly into the contours of the foot, so use it to make circular strokes, relaxing the sole, sides, arches, and instep.

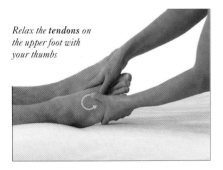

Relax the **tendons** *on the upper foot with your thumbs*

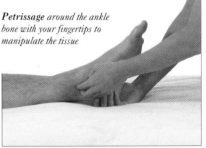

Petrissage *around the ankle bone with your fingertips to manipulate the tissue*

THE UPPER FOOT
Support the foot with your fingers, and massage thoroughly over the top of the foot, using your thumbs in small, alternate circles. Work up in parallel lines from toes to ankle.

THE ANKLE BONES
Slightly raise the foot and stroke around the outer ankle bone with your fingertips. Then make tiny circles close to the bone, one spot at a time. Repeat on the inner ankle bone.

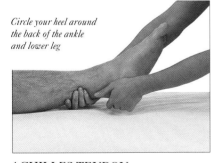

Circle your heel around the back of the ankle and lower leg

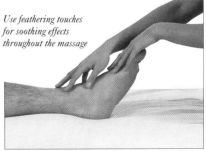

Use feathering touches for soothing effects throughout the massage

ACHILLES TENDON
Keep the foot raised and supported with one hand, while massaging around the sides and back of the heel with the heel of your hand. Focus particularly on the Achilles **tendon**.

FEATHERING STROKES
Rest the foot on the mattress and feather softly down with your fingertips, from ankle to toes, several times. This gives pleasurable relaxation as you continue your foot massage.

SKILL
12

FEET AND LOWER LEG

*Continuing to work on specific areas of the foot,
and making a connection with the leg*

THE TOES

A suprising amount of tension builds
up in the toes, as we tend to clench
them unconsciously when under
stress, or because our body weight
is unevenly distributed. The passive
movement and massage of each toe
ensure a release of tension, which has
a positive effect on the whole body.

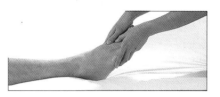

RELAXING THE TENDONS
Supporting the foot with one hand, slide your
thumb steadily along the grooves between
each **tendon**, from the base of the toes. Swop
hands to work on the outer side of the foot.

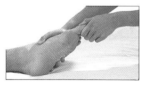

PULLING TOES
Hold the foot with one hand,
and pull each toe from base to
tip between your thumb and
forefinger, squeezing the tip.

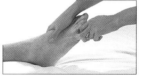

STROKING TOES
Clasp each toe at the base,
between your forefinger and
middle finger, and draw them
along, stroking the sides.

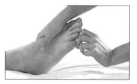

WIGGLING TOES
Grasp the end of each toe
and wiggle it up and down.
Rotate the toe gently, and
then squeeze all along it.

THE SOLE

*Always put your whole
attention into your
touch, even if your
hand is motionless*

Uncomfortable shoes and prolonged
standing cramp the complex structure
of the foot, so that **ligaments** and
muscles become tense. By massaging
the soles of the feet, you can alleviate
tension, disperse toxins back into the
lymphatic drainage system, and
revitalize the whole blood supply.

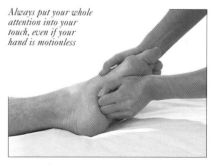

*Sink your thumb pad in
slowly so that the tissue
softens under its weight*

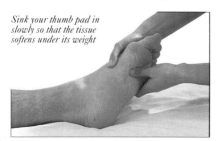

KNUCKLE STRETCH
Above: Supporting the top of the foot, use
the flat edge of your knuckles to stretch the
thick layer of skin covering the sole, from the
outer edge of the heel to the base of the toes.

THUMB PRESSURE
Left: Apply a steady pressure over the entire
sole, one point at a time. When you think you
have reached the right depth, rotate your
thumb on the spot and then slowly withdraw.

THE ANKLE

There are seven bones in the ankle. These bear the entire weight of the body when it is in motion. Running behind the ankle is the Achilles **tendon**, the strongest in the body. At the front of the ankle, a thick band of **ligaments** binds the tendons of the muscles responsible for moving the foot. Massage and passive movement will help to keep the area supple.

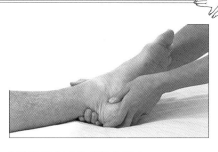

PETRISSAGE STROKES
Support the ankle with one hand, and use your other thumb to make **petrissage** strokes all around the sides of the heel and ankle.

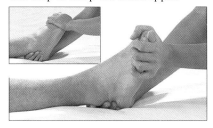

ROTATE THE ANKLE
Slowly rotate the ankle joint three times, both ways. Then flex and extend the foot to stretch the **ligaments** and Achilles **tendon**.

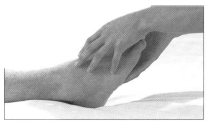

FEATHERING FINISH
Using the tips of your fingers, feather lightly down from the lower leg, over the sole of the foot, and out of the toes for a delightful finish.

MASSAGING THE LEG

After massaging the foot, you will want to continue on the leg. Spread oil downwards and then apply **main strokes** (see p.41) to integrate the whole limb. Boost the circulation with upward flowing fanning strokes. Use kneading (pp.50-51) and **petrissage** (pp.54-55) on the front of the leg and finish with stroking, feathering, and connection holds. Massage the other foot and leg, and complete with a hold on both feet for balance and rest.

CONNECTION

Make a connection hold between the ankle and knee to ensure the joints are warm and relaxed. Passive movements on the leg (p.35) will loosen the hip and knee, helping your partner to release its weight into your hands.

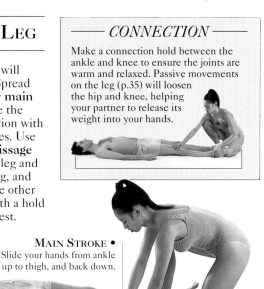

MAIN STROKE •
Slide your hands from ankle up to thigh, and back down.

SKILL

13 COMPLETING THE SESSION

DAY 2

Definition: *Creating the perfect finish to a relaxing massage*

IT IS IMPORTANT to complete your session with as much care as you took over the initial stages. You must allow your partner some time to absorb the benefits of the session. If you move away too abruptly, he may feel abandoned, since he will have become accustomed to the contact of your touch. Leave your partner snug and warm, so that he can relax for about five minutes. After helping your partner to his feet, take the time to thank each other.

OBJECTIVE: To leave your partner feeling good. *Rating* ••

Step 1
FINAL HOLD

Before practising this final skill, make a series of **energy balancing** holds. Then place your hands on the feet, or around the crown of the head. Close your eyes to focus your attention on your partner for at least a minute, and withdraw your hands slowly.

BOTH FEET •
Clasp both feet in this **energy balancing** hold, bringing a restful sense of balance.

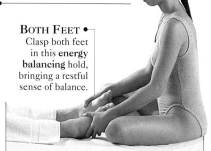

Step 2
TIME TO RELAX

COVER UP •
Explain to your partner that you are covering him up and he can now relax, or he may feel obliged to start getting up.

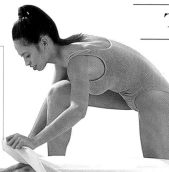

Now cover your partner with a large towel or warm sheet, so that he can relax for some minutes without becoming chilled. You may want to keep a blanket close by if you are concerned about the temperature.

Step 3
ABSORB THE EFFECTS

Allow time to assimilate the effects of
the massage. Your partner may feel
vulnerable, as a result of releasing
physical and emotional tension, and
you will need to relax any tension
that you have accumulated, and
to rest. After some moments,
leave to wash your hands.

CARING TOUCH
Massage is sometimes
called a language of
love, for its quality of
caring conveys the
essence of healing.
Bring the session to a
perfect conclusion by
sitting silently, your
hands resting gently on
your partner's body.

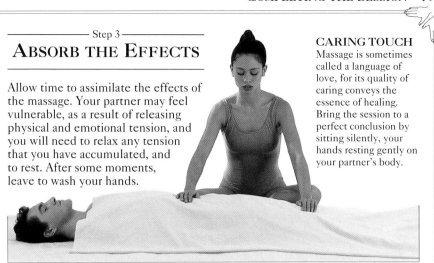

Steps 4 & 5
HELPING UP

Sometimes people become so relaxed
in massage that they have difficulty in
re-orienting themselves immediately
afterwards. At other times, they may
bounce off the mattress energetically.
Be there to guide your partner back
to his feet, focusing his attention on
his body so that he feels stable and
grounded. Spend some time talking
about the session, and thank your
partner for letting you massage him.

SHARE THANKS
This is a good time to
thank each other for
the equally important
aspects of giving and
receiving,
which has
made this
experience
possible.

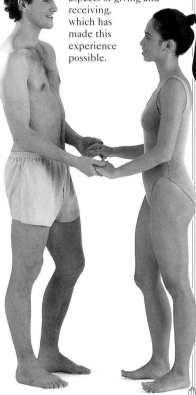

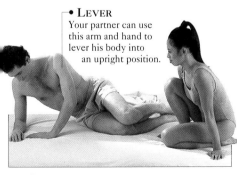

• LEVER
Your partner can use
this arm and hand to
lever his body into
an upright position.

GETTING UP
It is a common habit to put a strain on the back
muscles when getting up from a lying position.
This can immediately undo your good work.
Tell your partner to turn on his side, drawing
in his knees, ready to lever his body upwards.

AFTER THE WEEKEND

Improving on your new techniques

DURING THE WEEKEND you have learnt a range of different massage techniques, and by now you will know how, when, and where to apply them. You should be feeling much more confident in your hands, and eager to start practising and combining the strokes into a full body massage. It is natural, when you first learn these skills, to concentrate purely on trying to get the movements and holds exactly right. You will then want to progress towards a flowing and caring massage that acknowledges the whole person with whom you are working – a massage that evokes beneficial changes in body, mind, and emotions – and touches the "**being**" level of your partner. You must trust in your intuitive responses and feelings, and there is no better way to do this than to practise massage as much as possible. Offer to work on family, friends, and colleagues, and invite them to give you constructive criticism. When you are comfortable with all your techniques, you can start massaging in a less academic, and more instinctive way. Touch is a natural expression of healing and communication between human beings, once we give ourselves permission to trust our hands.

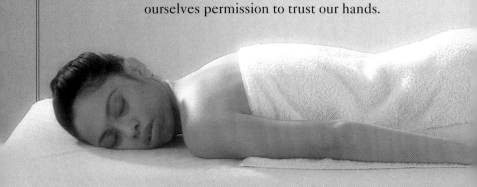

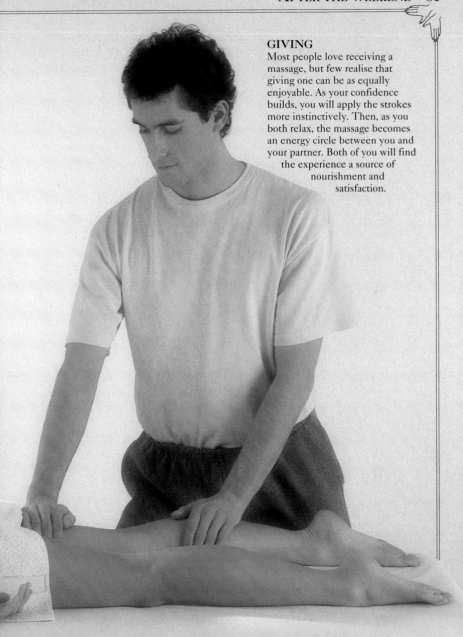

GIVING

Most people love receiving a massage, but few realise that giving one can be as equally enjoyable. As your confidence builds, you will apply the strokes more instinctively. Then, as you both relax, the massage becomes an energy circle between you and your partner. Both of you will find the experience a source of nourishment and satisfaction.

FULL BODY MASSAGE

How to create a flowing sequence of strokes for a whole body massage

THIS SEQUENCE OF STROKES shows you how to combine all that you have learnt. Here it is suggested that you begin your massage on the back of the body, and complete it on the front as this is a comfortable way for you both to build up trust. However, once you feel confident, start the massage wherever you feel is appropriate, and maintain a flowing and harmonious sequence.

BACK OF BODY

Welcome your partner and help him to settle comfortably on the mattress. Cover with a sheet, and begin with a connection hold so that you both can relax into the contact of touch. Apply **postural** ease strokes to the shoulders, pelvic area, and legs. This massage will start on the back. Apply oil only to the area you are about to massage.

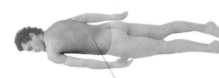

SOOTHE THE BACK •
Position yourself above the head. After three **main strokes**, follow up with fanning and other effleurage strokes. Stretch the area alongside the spine with thumb pressure **petrissage** strokes. From the side of the body, apply all the different effleurage movements, until you feel the whole surface of the back relaxing.

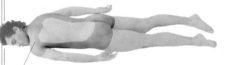

• KNEAD THE BACK
Knead the fleshy areas of the buttocks, the sides of the back, under the shoulder blades, over the shoulders, and base of the neck on the opposite side from you. Swop sides, and work thoroughly over the same areas on the other side. Follow up kneading with soothing effleurage strokes.

• PETRISSAGE ON THE BACK
Using the heels of hands, thumb pads and fingertips, go deeper with **petrissage** strokes over the **sacrum**, up alongside the spine, around the shoulder blades, and shoulders. Connect the whole back with several full **main strokes**, and finish by feathering the skin lightly.

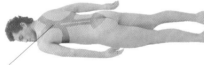

THE CALF
Connect the **sacrum** or hip, and the foot of the leg you are about to massage, with a hold. Start with three **main strokes** moving up from the ankle to encompass the whole leg, buttocks, and pelvic area. Apply effleurage, kneading, and **petrissage** to the lower leg, focusing on the calf area. Complete with a main stroke of the whole leg.

• THE THIGH
Continue with your strokes on the back and sides of the upper leg area. Once the muscles have relaxed with soothing effleurage strokes, knead the fleshy region of the thigh and then follow up with **petrissage**. Integrate with a full **main stroke** over the whole leg. Connect the two sides of the body by holding the soles of both feet, and repeat all your strokes on the other leg.

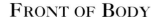

-COMPLETE THE BACK-

To complete the back of the body massage, apply **percussion** movements (cupping, hacking, or pummelling), working upwards over fleshy areas such as the calf, thigh, buttocks, and around the shoulders. Only apply these strokes if you want to bring a stimulatory effect to the massage at this point. Finish by feathering down the whole body.

FRONT OF BODY

Ask your partner to turn over to lie on his back, and cover him with a sheet. Apply **postural** ease movements to the neck, shoulders and arms, and on hips and legs in the lower body. Give an **energy balancing** hold while he settles into the new position.

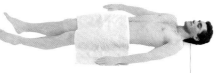

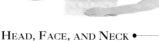

HEAD, FACE, AND NECK •

Position yourself above your partner's head. Begin with passive movements – lifting and rolling the head to ease tension from the neck, and then follow the sequence of strokes from "Massage for Stress Relief" (see pp.60-63).

CHEST •

Make a connection hold, and apply oil to the chest, to start with three full **main strokes**. After fan strokes, follow up with kneading, and then **petrissage**, particularly on the pectoral muscles. Complete with a full **main stroke**.

THE BELLY •

Change position and move to the side of the body, to place your hands over heart and lower belly, to allow the abdominal area to relax. Start with slow, gentle circular motions on the belly, and continue with other soothing movements. Follow strokes for the belly from the "Working On Sensitive Areas" session, (see pp.66-69), and complete with a calming hold.

THE ARMS AND HANDS •

Make a connection hold between your partner's shoulder and hand. After passive movements, apply oil to the arm. Use your sequence of **main strokes**, effleurage, kneading, and **petrissage** on the lower arm, around the elbow, and over the upper arm. Make a full main stroke over the whole arm, then massage the hand (pp.72-73). Repeat the strokes on the other arm and hand.

—— COMPLETION ——

As with the back of the body, decide if revitalizing **percussion** strokes are appropriate now. You can use them over fleshy areas of the legs and arms on the front of the body. Once you have finished the massage, cover your partner with a sheet, and follow the procedures for "Completing A Massage" (see pp.78-79).

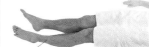

• LEGS AND FEET

Begin with a connection hold to integrate upper and lower body joints. Apply oil to the leg, and make three full **main strokes**. Massage the foot (see pp.76-77). Now proceed to massage the leg, starting with the ankle, shin, and knee, using effleurage, kneading, and **petrissage**. Repeat the sequence of strokes on the thigh area. Finish the leg massage with a complete **main stroke** and feathering downwards lightly. Repeat all your strokes on the other leg and foot.

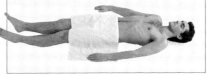

DEVELOPING TACTILE SENSES

How to heighten your awareness and sensitivity of touch

TOUCH IS THE FIRST SENSE experienced by a baby within the womb, as it explores its own developing body. Later in life, touch becomes the bridge between our inner selves and the world that surrounds us. The human brain is capable of registering, and responding to, a variety of tactile information, transmitted through the thousands of nerve endings in the hands. The more you develop your sense of touch, the deeper and better your massage will be. Hands not only channel energy, they receive messages from the body about how to touch, where to touch, and how deep to touch. This is the intuitive level of massage, which combined with your techniques, can make massage such a profound and healing work. These exercises will help you to bring a heightened awareness to your hands and your tactile senses.

LEARNING TO TOUCH

Focus your attention on your hands and set yourself exercises where you bring all your awareness to the sensations imparted by whatever you are touching or holding. Try to recapture the wonder of touch that you must have experienced in the first years of childhood. This will increase both your sensitivity and perception in massage.

FINGERTIPS •
Delicately stroke your fingertips over your skin, tracing the bone structure of your face beneath them.

MOULDING HANDS
If you hold a smooth, round object, like a cup or bowl, let your hands melt into the curves, like a potter's hands moulding into clay.

TOUCHING YOUR SKIN
Explore the sensuality of touch by stroking your own body. Feel the smoothness of your skin and the variations in its temperature.

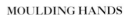

EXPLORING TEXTILES

Certain textiles have a luxurious and soothing feel against the skin. By touching a range of different materials, you will begin to enhance your sensory awareness. The delicate gossamer of chiffon, the comforting richness of velvet, and the light caress of silk can all expand your sense of touch as you play with them.

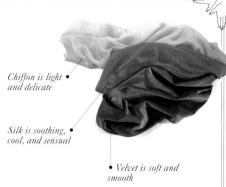

Chiffon is light • and delicate

Silk is soothing, • cool, and sensual

• Velvet is soft and smooth

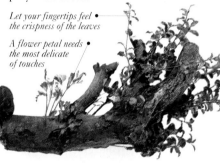

Let your fingertips feel • the crispness of the leaves

A flower petal needs • the most delicate of touches

NATURAL TEXTURES

Nature is rich in texture. We commonly use sight, sound, and smell to take in nature's essence, so now include your tactile senses. Fragile flower petals, rugged fallen logs, and the delicate tendrils of emerging leaves all elicit different types of touching response from you.

MAN-MADE SHAPES

Man-made objects can be constructed from a variety of materials such as clay, stone, steel, wood, rubber, and modelling clay, and fall into round, rectangular, hard and soft, utensils, tools, or toys. As you pick up various objects, focus on how your hands hold or grip each item, and their heat or cold, and density, or pliability.

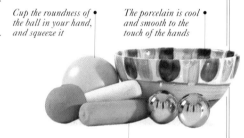

Cup the roundness of • the ball in your hand, and squeeze it

The porcelain is cool • and smooth to the touch of the hands

The pliability of modelling clay • brings suppleness to your hands

FLEXIBILITY EXERCISES

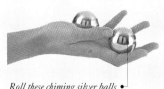

Roll these chiming silver balls • around one hand at a time to increase the suppleness and energy of your touch

Like any tools of the trade, your hands should be in good condition. In terms of giving massage, this means suppleness of movement, flexibility in the joints, warmth, and a lightness of touch. Exercising your hands regularly will help to keep them fit. To increase hand dexterity and co-ordination, try simple juggling, kneading dough or modelling clay, and squeezing pliable or rubbery objects. These silver balls, left, called Shou Xing, are originally from Chinese healing traditions, and as you play with them, the chimes resonate to relax the mind.

SHARING YOUR SKILL

How to share your massage skills in quick and easy ways

THERE ARE MANY OCCASIONS when a friend could benefit from your massage skills. Sometimes a quick massage is sufficient to ease tense muscles, or revitalize a tired or sluggish system. You might be called upon to share your skills with colleagues at work, at a social event, or when a visiting friend. This sequence shows you how to bring relief to the shoulders, neck, and head, which are usually the main areas of tension. While giving this massage, check that your own **posture** remains relaxed.

STROKES TO RELAX

After soft strokes over the shoulders and down the back, relax shoulder and neck muscles with kneading, **petrissage**, and **percussion**. Start by resting both hands over the shoulders for a few moments.

SQUEEZE THE SHOULDERS
Above: Clasp the front of the shoulders with your fingers to knead across the shoulders, by lifting and squeezing the **trapezius muscles**.

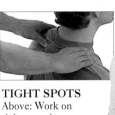

TIGHT SPOTS
Above: Work on tight spots between the shoulder blades with your thumb pads, wherever you find **uric acid** granules.

KNEADING THE ARMS
Above: Continue kneading down both arms to the elbows. Lift and squeeze the flesh all around the **biceps** and **triceps**.

EASE THE SPINE
Left: Make small **petrissage** rotations with your thumbs, along the top of the spine.

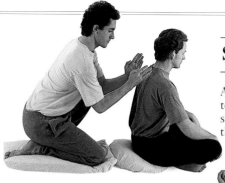

PERCUSSION

Cupping and hacking, between the spine and the shoulder blades, work well from this position, to invigorate and release tension.

STIMULATING STROKES

Any habitual pattern of **postural** tension will lead to a tightening of the shoulder muscles, causing stiffness in the neck, and constricting the blood circulation to the brain. Stimulate the area with vibrant **percussion**.

TONE-UP
Left: Pummelling over the shoulders tones up this area.

NECK RELEASE

Once the shoulders are loosened, turn your attention to the neck. Interlock your fingers and place your hands over the base of the neck. Scoop up the muscle by sliding your heels inwards with firm but careful pressure. Release, and work up to the top of the neck.

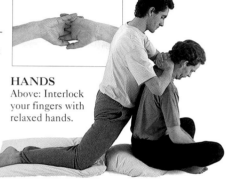

HANDS
Above: Interlock your fingers with relaxed hands.

• SPINE
Help your friend to lengthen his spine.

HEAD FORWARD
Ask your friend to bend his head slightly forward in order to knead the neck muscles.

EXTEND THE SPINE
Left: From the abdomen and the base of the spine, draw your hands slowly upwards.

• FOREARMS
Keep your elbows flexed and your wrists relaxed.

FINISHING TOUCH

Finally, make **petrissage** rotations over the whole scalp with the fingertips on both of your hands. Feel the thin layer of muscle slide about over the skull. Then briskly rub your fingertips all over the head to create friction against the scalp. Draw tension away from the whole area by stroking your fingers out of the hair.

POSTURE •
Ensure your shoulders are relaxed and your spine straight, while massaging your friend.

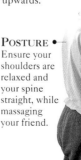
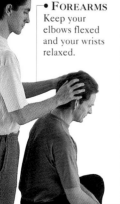

INCREASING YOUR POTENTIAL

How to improve your skills and become professional at massage

---

MOST PEOPLE LEARN HOW TO MASSAGE because it is a caring skill which can be shared with family or friends. Once you have mastered the basic techniques, and become relaxed and confident in giving your massage, you may want to improve your skills, and even consider acquiring professional status as a massage therapist. Massage is an exciting world, with wide possibilities of increasing your breadth of knowledge in the field of healthcare. You can enhance your massage skills by studying complementary subjects, such as **aromatherapy**, deep tissue massage, or **reflexology**, which concentrates on the feet. Here are some straightforward suggestions to help you improve your status as a massage therapist: taking further training, gaining a professional diploma, improving your own body awareness, and acquiring a massage table.

TAKING A COURSE

To achieve professional status as a massage therapist, it is usually a requirement to have an approved diploma within the particular field that you intend to practise. This is achieved by studying in a recognized school, or with a qualified teacher, for a set number of hours. You must usually pass examinations in both the practical section, and in anatomy and **physiology** theory, although study requirements may vary locally.

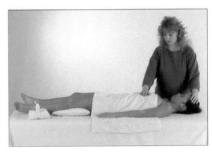

TAKING TRAINING
The advantages of joining massage training, is that you have the opportunity to watch a professional therapist at work, who can share their experience with you. You will be able to practise on fellow students, and to give each other valuable constructive criticism.

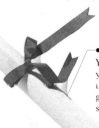

• DIPLOMA
You can display your diploma in the area where you give your massage sessions.

QUALIFICATION
Achieving a recognized qualification will be acknowledged by a certificate, allowing you to set up a professional practice. Even if you do not wish to turn professional, this will add to your confidence, and that of your friends.

RELATED DISCIPLINES

Anyone working in a therapeutic field should continue to improve on their own physical and psychological awareness. All physical exercise and relaxation techniques will bring a vitality and freshness to the quality of your massage. Understanding the principle of **holistic** care – that body and mind are linked – and disciplines such as Yoga and T'ai Chi, can prove valuable.

YOGA

Yoga originates from the spiritual traditions of India, and has become extremely popular in the West. There are different schools of Yoga, and the discipline works mainly through a series of body stretches, in conjunction with your breathing.

T'AI CHI CH'UAN

T'ai Chi is a Chinese martial art exercise that focuses particularly on meditation, stamina, **posture**, and motion. It is a complement to massage, for it teaches you flowing movement, and how to increase your vital life energy, or "chi".

POSTURE •

The **posture** and movement of T'ai Chi Ch'uan increases a stability and **grounding** in the body, that is essential in massage.

SEQUENCES

Each T'ai Chi motion is co-ordinated with your breathing, and throughout the shifts of movement, the focus is on the "hara", or **centre** of stillness within your belly, from which all movement and "chi" arises.

BUYING A TABLE

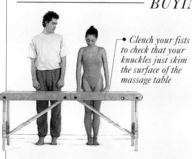

• *Clench your fists to check that your knuckles just skim the surface of the massage table*

CHECKING THE SIZE

A massage table should be at least 1.8m (6ft) long and about 0.6 to 0.8m (2 to 2½ft) wide. The correct height of a table should be level with the surface of your knuckles.

While some people are content to massage at floor level, most will find that working on a table adds to their comfort, and also improves their professional image. Buying or building a massage table is a worthwhile investment, and care should be given to selecting one that suits your needs. The table should be the right size, and sturdy enough to support not only your friend's weight, but also the pressure and movement you apply. There should be at least 2.5cm (1in) of foam padding on the surface, with a vinyl cover for easy cleaning. Fold-up tables can be stored readily, and if light enough, are portable when you visit clients in their own homes.

STANDING POSTURE

Taking care of your posture while standing

ONCE YOU ARE WORKING at a massage table, you will find it much easier to move around your partner's body. However, you still need to take good care of your **posture** to avoid straining your back muscles. The main principles of a good standing posture in massage are: firstly, to feel **grounded** and stable in the lower half of your body, by dropping your weight down through your pelvis, buttocks, and legs towards your feet and the ground. Secondly, you should lengthen your spine upwards, and keep your neck extended with your head balanced over the spinal column. Thirdly, let your shoulders be relaxed and wide, and your arms open and free from your body. Always bend forward from your hips, and keep your feet apart with your knees flexed, so that you can shift your balance from side to side.

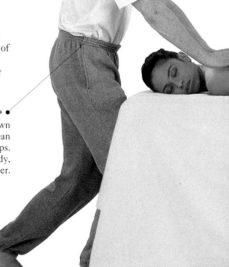

• HEAD
Remember to keep your head "floating upwards" to avoid strain on your neck muscles.

STAYING CENTRED
To stay fresh and energized while giving a massage, keep your **posture** easy and relaxed. Co-ordinate your movements with your breathing, and try to maintain a sense of moving from your **centre**. It is helpful to visualize that your source of vital energy, or centre, is located in the lower belly region.

BEND FROM THE HIP •
While making a long stroke down the body, particularly the back, lean forward by tilting from your hips. Avoid making contact with your body, or leaning too far over your partner.

YOUR FEET •
Keep your feet apart to provide balance and stability for your body, and to enable you to shift your weight back and forth as you make the strokes.

HOW NOT TO STAND

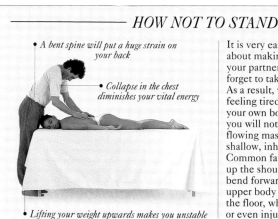

A bent spine will put a huge strain on your back

Collapse in the chest diminishes your vital energy

Lifting your weight upwards makes you unstable

It is very easy to become so concerned about making things comfortable for your partner, that you completely forget to take care of your own **posture**. As a result, you can finish a massage feeling tired, irritable, and tense. If your own body is not relaxed and open, you will not be able to give a fully flowing massage, as your breathing is shallow, inhibiting your vital energy. Common faults in posture are to hunch up the shoulders and hang the head, to bend forward, or to use the spine and upper body to lift your weight up off the floor, which can create pain, strain, or even injury to your back.

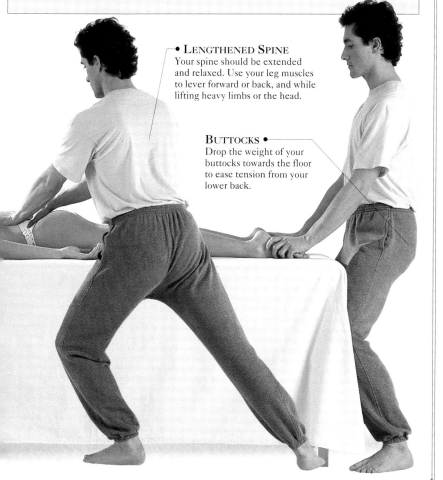

• LENGTHENED SPINE
Your spine should be extended and relaxed. Use your leg muscles to lever forward or back, and while lifting heavy limbs or the head.

BUTTOCKS •
Drop the weight of your buttocks towards the floor to ease tension from your lower back.

GLOSSARY

Words in *italic* are glossary entries.

A

• **Aromatherapy** The treatment of physical and emotional conditions by using aromatic *essential oils*.
• **Autonomic nervous system** The control of the involuntary, or non-conscious, action of smooth muscles, cardiac muscles, and glands. It has two divisions: the sympathetic and para-sympathetic systems. The sympathetic system responds to stress, enabling a person to react to danger by taking a "fight or flight" mode. The para-sympathetic does the opposite, slowing down bodily functions, allowing the body to rest and replenish its energy. Massage is believed to have a beneficial effect on the parasympathetic system.

B

• **Balancing** A term used in body therapy and applied to techniques that bring a sense of integration, harmony, balance or equilibrum to and within the body, mind, and emotions.
• **Being** The "being" quality is a concept of *holistic* massage, where the calm, still presence of the person giving or receiving the massage is considered as important as the "doing" aspect of the techniques or strokes, particularly in *energy balancing* work.
• **Biceps** The muscle bulk at the front of the upper arm, which flexes the forearm, and rotates it outwards.

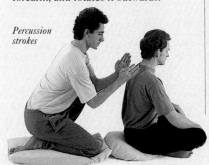

Percussion strokes

• **Breath flow** The awareness of breath as important in massage. Full breathing increases energy and stamina.

C

• **Carrier oil** The basic oil used as a lubricant in massage.
• **Centre** A term used in bodywork, meditation, therapeutic, and martial art techniques referring to the individual's source of life-force energy. To be centred is to be at peace with oneself.
• **Central nervous system** The mass of nerve tissue which makes up the brain and the spinal column, receiving and analyzing information, and transmitting appropriate instructions.
• **Circulatory system** The heart, blood vessels and blood, and the *lymphatic* system. It carries oxygen and nutrients to cells and tissues, and removes carbon dioxide and waste.

E

• **Energy balancing** A technique to calm and create a sense of equilibrium within the body, and mind of the person receiving massage, by the simple "laying of hands".
• **Essential oil** Aromatic essences derived from plants, herbs, and flowers. These are blended with oils and used for their healing properties.
• **External oblique muscles** Muscles of the abdominal wall that contract to bend the *vertebral column*.

G

• **Grounding** The concept of creating a sense of stability, equilibrium, and support in the body, mind, and emotions. On a physical level, it means bringing an awareness to the centre of gravity in the body, which is located in the pelvic region. To be emotionally grounded is to feel safe, secure, and in touch with reality.
• **Gluteals** The large muscles of the buttocks. Unique to humans, they straighten the hip, allowing us to stand erect, and control thigh movement.

H

• **Holistic** The integral relationship between body, mind, emotions, and spirit. In massage, it means the focus is on all aspects of the whole person.
• **Humerus** The long bone of the upper arm, from shoulder to elbow.

L

• **Ligaments** Elastic connective tissue which binds bone to bone, and inhibits excessive movement of joints. It also supports internal organs.
• **Lymphatic system** A secondary *circulatory system* which drains lymph, a plasma-like fluid, from body tissue back into the bloodstream. It plays a major role in defence against disease by trapping foreign matter in the lymph nodes, and circulating white blood cells which fight infection. The system has no pump, so gravity and the movement of muscles force the flow of lymph around the body. Massage boosts this system, especially when directed towards the heart, or a lymph node.

M

• **Main stroke** A long effleurage stroke which encompasses the part of the body that is about to be massaged.

P

• **Pectoral muscles** Large muscles of the chest which lift and rotate the arm.
• **Percussion** A series of stimulating and revitalizing massage movements.
• **Petrissage** A deeper stroke that pushes muscle towards the bone, and helps to grind away waste products.
• **Physiology** The functioning of the various systems of the body.
• **Posture/Postural** The structure and balance of weight of different parts of the body in relationship to each other.

R

• **Radius** The shorter of the two long bones of the forearm, it runs from the elbow to the wrist on the thumb side.
• **Reflexology** A system of treating body disorders by applying pressure to specific parts of the feet. Also known as zone therapy, these points are believed to correspond directly with different parts of the body.

S

• **Sacrum** The triangular bone at the base of the spine in the pelvic girdle, formed by the fusion of five *vertebrae*.
• **Soft tissue** Tissue surrounding the body's skeleton, including muscles, *tendons*, and *ligaments*.

T

• **Tendons** Fibrous tissue that attaches muscle to bone, or muscle to muscle.
• **Thorax/Thoracic cavity** The chest area containing the lungs and heart, which is protected by the ribcage.
• **Trapezius muscle** A large, diamond-shaped muscle that runs across the upper back. It is involved in raising the arm, supporting the spine and neck, and extending the head.
• **Triceps muscle** The muscle that runs along the back of the upper arm. It extends the elbow and forearm.

U

• **Ulna** One of the two long bones of the forearm, it runs from elbow to wrist on the side of the little finger.
• **Uric acid** A waste product excreted during muscular activity, and if trapped will cause feelings of stiffness. It is carried by the blood and *lymphatic* systems to the kidneys for elimination.

V

• **Vertebrae/Vertebral column** The spine, or vertebral column, consists of 33 bones called vertebrae. It protects the spinal cord, from which nerves run to all parts of the body. The spine gives support to the upper half of the body, and provides attachment for the ribs and muscles of the back.

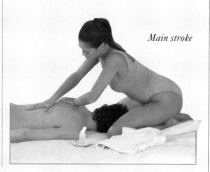

Main stroke

INDEX

GETTING IN TOUCH

ITEC (International Therapy
Examination Council)
James House
Oakelbrook Mill
Newent
Gloucestershire GL18 1HD

AMPTE
(Association of Massage Practitioners
Training Executive)
24 Highbury Grove
London
N5 1EA

ACKNOWLEDGMENTS

Nitya Lacroix and Dorling Kindersley would like to thank the following for
their help in the production of this book:

Rokiah Yaman and Jonathan Stigwood, who were the patient models.
Laurence Henderson for additional modelling.
Sakina Bowhay for helpful information on aromatherapy, and Sudhir Borowij
of the School of Holistic Massage, whose support and advice is always
appreciated. Also, Ian Guinan for anatomical information. The staff at
Stocks House, Tring, Hertfordshire, for the room location used in the book.

Jo Foord, photographer, and her assistant, Andy Adams. Jenny Jordan and
Emma Koch for hair and make-up. Sarah Larter for additional editorial
assistance, and Hilary Bird for the index. Janos Marffy and Simone End
for colour illustrations and line drawings, Alison Donovan and
Claire Pegrum for additional artwork. Location photography by
Philip Gatward, and his assistant, Jeremy Hopley (p.11tr).

A note from the Author: I would like to express my thanks to the editorial and
art team at Dorling Kindersley, particularly Liz Wheeler, Alison Donovan,
Jo Weeks, and Amanda Lunn.
Nitya Lacroix and Sudhir Borowij are co-directors of the London and
Surrey-based School of Holistic Massage. For details, write to:
School of Holistic Massage, 26 Old Barn View, Bargate,
Godalming, Surrey GU7 1YR.

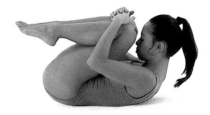